AF559938

TEACHING OF SOCIAL STUDIES

TEACHING OF SOCIAL STUDIES

A.S. KOHLI

ANMOL PUBLICATIONS PVT. LTD.
NEW DELHI - 110 002 (INDIA)

ANMOL PUBLICATIONS PVT. LTD.
Regd. Office: 4360/4, Ansari Road, Daryaganj,
New Delhi-110002 (India)
Tel.: 23278000, 23261597, 23286875, 23255577
Fax: 91-11-23280289
Email: anmolpub@gmail.com
Visit us at: www.anmolpublications.com

Branch Office: No. 1015, Ist Main Road, BSK IIIrd Stage
IIIrd Phase, IIIrd Block, Bengaluru-560 085 (India)
Tel.: 080-41723429 • Fax: 080-26723604
Email: anmolpublicationsbangalore@gmail.com

Teaching of Social Studies

First Published, 1996

Reprint, 1999, 2002, 2003, 2004, 2005, 2006, 2007, 2008, 2012, 2014

PRINTED IN INDIA

Printed at Balaji Offset Press, Delhi

Preface

This book is likely to serve a dual purpose i.e. a text book for prospective teachers in India and some other South-east Asian countries, who are looking forward for teaching of social studies in schools and a reference book to the practising teachers. The book will help the students to understand the aims, objectives, techniques and methods used for teaching of social studies in schools. Each topic in the book has been divided into heads and sub-heads and the material has been presented in a proper sequence keeping in mind the examination requirements. The topics have been dealt with in all their details and an attempt has been made to present the matter in a comprehensive and lucid manner. An effort has been made to present latest ideas on the subject and to make the subject matter up-to-date.

It is hoped that the book will be appreciated by students and teachers alike. While preparing the book, material has been drawn from works of different authors, periodicals and journals and the author is indebted to all such persons and their publishers.

I would also like to express my sincere gratitude to a number of friends and colleagues who have given many valuable suggestions. I am also thankful to my publishers for bringing out this book in such a nice form.

Comments and suggestions for the improvement of the book will be gratefully accepted.

A. S. KOHLI

Contents

1

Meaning, Nature and Scope of Social Studies

1.1. INTRODUCTION

After Independence while deciding the aim of our educational system it was expected our institutions to contribute directly to the development of good citizenship, loyalty to democracy, civic responsibility and human relationship. They should also help the youth of the day to prepare themselves for well adjusted lives in the twenty-first century. To achieve these objectives it was expected that our schools will help the students to acquire a philosophy of life, attitudes, skills, concepts, understanding and knowledge that is useful to them for next 5-6 decades. In attainment of these aims of education, the study of social studies as an independent field of study is quite important.

1.2. WHAT IS SOCIAL STUDIES?

"Social Studies" is a school subject that deals with the human relationship. In America the use of the term human relationship started around the year 1916, however in India it is of recent origin.

We have witnessed various advances in science and technology during the previous 70-80 years which have helped to solve various problems of the mankind. However, they have also created a large number of problems which cannot be solved easily. In the process the greatest sufferer has been the system of human relationship that was built up on centuries of experience and great tradition. In this age of science and technology when the space travel is a reality the child finds himself in a rapidly changing and complex world. He is faced with one or the other type of problems and it is expected from schools that they prepare the child to deal intelligently with all such problems. To achieve this goal, the schools have to select the design their curriculum in such a way that it preserves the best from the past in terms of tradition and conduct and also teach children the application of the same in the modern age of science and technology. In order to achieve these, the field of social studies developed as an independent field of study in our secondary schools.

In social studies we deal with man and his interaction with his fellow beings and with his surroundings and environment. Thus social studies deals with man's relationship with his social and physical environment. The main aim of social studies is the development of a well informed, intelligent person capable of solving his day to day problems and keen to accept responsibility as a good citizen of the country having desirable and essential qualities required in a democratic society.

1.3. MISUNDERSTANDING ABOUT SOCIAL STUDIES

Though the teaching of social studies was introduced 30-40 years back yet there is a lot of misunderstanding about the scope of the subject even today. Teachers feel that social studies is nothing but a combination of History, Geography, Civics, Economics, Sociology etc. This misconception is supported by the subject-matter of existing text books on social studies and the methods adopted to teach the subject-matter. It is not an exaggeration to say that the situation has worsened. The confusion arises because of the fact that different sections of a textbook of social studies give detailed accounts of different social sciences unrelatedly. The teacher also teaches either pure history or a pure geography lesson and never a lesson on social studies.

For a common man social studies relates to social problems or current events. Though both these form an important part of social studies but they are not the only contents of the social studies. Social studies in addition to the social problems and current events also deals with physical, social and cultural environment of man. However, it must be very clearly understood that social studies is not a combination of different social sciences, nor it is only a social problem or current events.

1.4. CORRECT CONCEPT AND NATURE OF SOCIAL STUDIES

It has been amply made clear in the previous section that social studies is not a combination of history, geography, civics etc. and that it is an independent field of study. It deals with the "study of relations and inter-relations--historical, geographical and social--and it provides the young mind the basis of public knowledge and orientation to life. In the absence of such a knowledge he will not be able to develop an integrated personality, he will not be able to tap his energies etc." A study of social studies enables the child to know about past and present and to establish a relationship between them. This knowledge of past and present relates to various fields of knowledge including local and distant, and personal and native lives, and also the lives and cultures of other men and women from different parts of the world. In any social studies course, there is always the material that "provides a core of knowledge, experience and insight around which other subjects; at whatever degree of specialization, may be built up in a coordinated way."

Basically social studies aims that each future generation grasps the necessary information about the social conditions that surround it and faster the requisite social attitudes and skills that enable young men and women to be effective members of a society in the changing world. Another point on which teachers must emphasize is that the attitudes, skills and understandings which helped our fore-fathers in survival and success in life may not be sufficient for the survival and success of the present generation.

Writing about the true concept of social studies, the Social Studies Committee of Schools Board Victoria (USA), in its publication "Social Studies for Schools" observes, what we study in social studies, is the life of a man in some particular place, at some particular time, we therefore, use every possible "subject". to help us understanding his problems and how he dealt or deals with them. The main aim is to give a better understanding of present problems. We try to give our future citizens some true understanding of the development of mankind. We attempt to trace with the children the fascinating story of how man has developed through the ages, of how man has studied to use and control his environment and how his life has been influenced by this, how our institutions have grown out of the past and should, therefore, be respected and how they have undergone many changes to meet changing needs and must undergo many more from time to time. Man's struggle with his environment yesterday and today, man's use of his powers and resources, his development, the essential unity of civilization, these are the main themes of Social Studies. We are trying to break the habit of putting knowledge into water-tight compartments, labelled history, geography, civics, economics etc. We are also trying to train children in the habits of thinking clearly, to be able to use all the knowledge at their command to solve problems and to be able to find the necessary information."

In the words of J.F. Forrester, "Social Studies, as the very name suggests, is the study of society and its chief aim is to help pupils to understand the world in which they have to live and how it came to be, so that they may become responsible citizens. It aims at promoting critical thinking and a readiness for social change, at creating a disposition for acting on behalf of the general welfare, at an appreciation of other cultures and a realization of the interdependence of man and man and of nation and nation."

The Secondary Education Commission of the National Education Association USA has defined Social Studies as follows:

"Social Studies are understood to be those whose subject-matter relates directly to the organisation and development of human society and to man as a member of social group." In the words of M.P. Muffatt, a person may be learned in Chemistry or Mathematics; he may be a skilled technician. But if he is shortsighted in his attitude to his fellow-men, he is unsocial and perhaps ill-adjusted in many other ways. The art of living is a fine art to which Social Studies contributes understanding.

The Report of Secondary Education Commission in India, has clearly stated: "Social Studies, as a term is comparatively new in Indian Education. It is meant to cover the ground, traditionally associated with History, Geography, Economics, Civics etc. If the teaching of these separate subjects only imparts *miscellaneous* and unrelated information and does not throw any light on or provide insight into social conditions and problems or create the desire to improve the existing state of things, their educative significance will be negligible. This whole group of studies has therefore, to be viewed as a compact whole whose object is to adjust the students to their social environment which includes the family, community, state and nation -- so that they may be able to understand how society has come to its present form. They may be able to interpret intelligently by matrix of social forces and movement in the midst of which they are living. This subject should help the students to discover and explain how this adjustment has taken place in the past and how it is taking place today. Through this subject the students should be able to acquire not only the knowledge but attitudes and values which are essential for successful group living and civics efficiency. It should endeavour to give the students not only a sense of national patriotism and an appreciation of national heritage, but also a keen and lively sense of world unity and world citizenship."

From the above discussion it becomes clear that social studies lay more stress on formation of standards, attitudes, ideals and interests in comparison to the imparting of factual knowledge. It helps in real intellectual advancement by providing knowledge with experience. It helps to integrate the knowledge of all social sciences and because of this it is sometimes called "coordinated and coordinating" by nature.

Thus both the words "social" and "studies" are quite important in terms of "Social Studies." It emphasizes that the study must be "social" i.e., a study **of** society, **for** society and **through** society. It is a study of society both in time and space. It deals with the study of the development of various social institutions such as family, caste system, marriage, governance etc.

It is a study **for** the improvement of society. It is expected that the child will bring about some improvement in the society by his contribution. It is a study **through** the society as the practical knowledge in this subject is provided through actual participation in the activities of society to which the child belongs. Though child is taught about the society in other subjects as well but each subject deals with a particular aspect of man and his natural environment. Social studies deals with man from all angles. In social studies we expect that the present generation of pupils will become better individuals and more effective members of the various groups in which they function.

The subject includes elements of geography, history, sociology, political science, economics, anthropology and other allied fields. It also draws material from all the social sciences, relating to the study of human relationships, human institutions and human behaviour. But in doing so, undue emphasis is not laid on any one subject or part, at the cost of another. Historical elements, for example, are studied objectively so that appreciation of the past may help to understand the present and anticipate the future. This means that the topics selected for study in social studies will not be limited to any particular subject. In the process of study, there will be a natural movement into many fields, if in any way, it can help in the solution of human problems and understanding of the human society and human relationships.

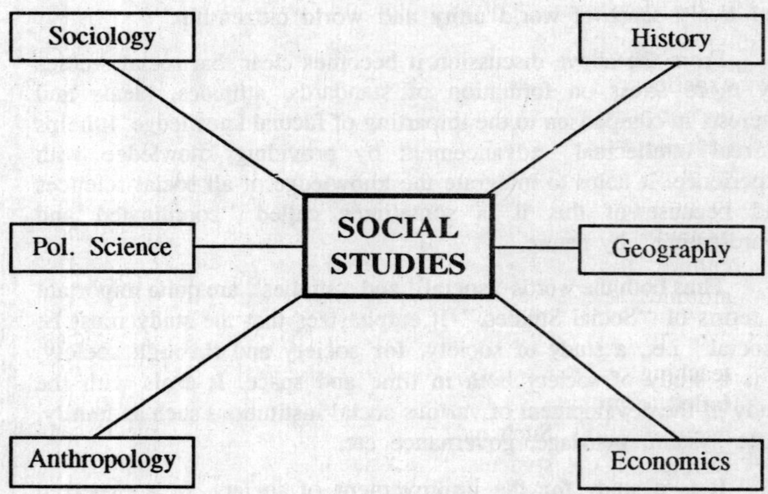

In the changing scenario of educational programmes we find the emphasis is being laid on teaching the subjects in an interrelated manner and it is in the fitness of things that a unified course of social studies be taught instead of separate subjects of history, geography, civics etc. The course in social studies for teaching as secondary stage may include topics from these subjects. The topics selected should be such as to introduce the young child to his physical and social environment. The reasons advanced against teaching of these subjects at the secondary level are as follows:

The knowledge given in isolation in various subjects cannot be easily understood and grasped by the students as the students are not interested in disconnected ideas offered by a number of subjects.

It is better if only a few important ideas with all possible combinations are given as it would put less burden on the children.

The aim of education at the secondary stage is to impart only a general and liberal education. Since for a large number of students it may be the final and conclusive stage of education so we should aim at widening their vision and outlook on life as a whole. It would help them to play an effective part as useful and democratic citizens. This is achieved in a better way by teaching them social studies because it not only includes knowledge of physical, cultural, economic, social and civic experiences of man but also includes in it the development of attitudes and skills.

Since the community life that provided the child with rich experiences previously has now become more complex and the home do not provide that awareness of relationship which was done in the past. Because of changed circumstances the schools are now required to provide what home and community provided in the past. "It has to provide total education -- education for knowledge, for background, for standards for awareness, for skills, for understanding for culture, for making a contribution, for a sense of belonging, for attitudes and for a proper orientation of modern world."

It can be easily achieved by teaching social studies. The teaching of separate subjects such as history, geography, civics, etc. failed to provide an integrated knowledge of the social problems of every day life. Such individualised study of the subjects cannot be utilized by the students to acquaint themselves with the immediate problems of nation, society or world that influence their daily life and thus it does not help them in solving the problems of daily life.

The study of each subject deals with only a limited scope concerning their field but in modern complex society the entire outlook has to be changed. It is now desirable that we start with the present day life of man and then see the extent to which he has learnt to control or be controlled by his physical environments. It can be achieved only through a unified course of social studies because the process of synthesizing these subjects into one field will remove the limitations of each subject.

Also to create a more enlightened citizenry, which is the need of the hour, we should provide knowledge in an integrated form instead of isolated subjects. Our curricula should reflect current thought and should be integrated with actual problems of every day life. This type of curriculum is possible if we teach social studies instead of teaching separate subjects of history, geography, civics etc.

Another reason advanced for the teaching of social studies is removed in the words of Happold, "Much of the literature, our students read, much of history and geography they learn, they will soon forget, what of value will remain? The ability to read with sense, the ability to speak and write sensitively and precisely, the ability to collect, sift and arrange various sorts of material, the ability to use books as a source both of information and of aesthetic pleasure, and the habit to think clearly and logically, in short, the acquisition of certain tools of learning and of certain skills are essential for every child today." It is only the unified course of Social Studies, which through its content and methods, emphasizes and trains for such attitudes and skills. Hence it has an advantage over the formal disciplines of history, geography and civics etc.

It can thus be argued that a unified course of social studies at school stage will make specialization in different subjects very easy at a later stage. In this way social studies provides the foundation for the super structure of specialization.

Hence teaching of composite course of social studies at secondary stage will prove useful in comparison to teaching of history, geography, economics, civics etc. as separate subjects.

1.5. DIFFERENCES BETWEEN SOCIAL STUDIES AND SOCIAL SCIENCES

Though we use the terms social studies and social sciences as synonyms yet the two are quite different terms. The discussion that follows will make these differences clear.

Both social studies and social sciences are concerned with the study of human relationships but in social science the emphasis is laid on research, investigation, discovery and experimentation. Social Sciences deal with detailed and systematic study of human relationships. They are written for adults. They maintain a certain standard of scholarship and are therefore not understood by school children. However, social sciences provide a lot of knowledge and a social scientist is ever willing to add a little more of human knowledge through his research and enquiry.

Unlike social sciences, the material that constitutes social studies is primarily for use in secondary schools. It contains those portions of social sciences that have been selected and adapted for the school use. Thus *social studies is a simplified and reorganised form of social sciences.* In it the human relationship is dealt with at the level of the child and not at the adult level as was the case in social sciences.

Basically the difference between social science and social studies is not in *kind* but only in *level of difficulty.* In comparison to social science, the social studies "must be simple, easy, appealing, interesting and learnable."

Another distinction between the two is that social sciences constitute the theoretical part of human affairs whereas the social studies deals with the practical part of human relationships. To illustrate this difference let us take the case of political science and civics. We find that political science is an advanced, scholarly subject that is taught and studied at depth in degree classes whereas civics is a simplified form of political science and is taught and studied in schools upto higher secondary standard.

The above discussion makes it quite clear that social sciences are those subjects which relate to the origin, organization, development of human society whereas social studies is concerned with those learning experiences that can easily be identified to have been drawn from social sciences in accordance with the needs of the school children.

While studying we study social sciences as separate subjects but we study social studies as an integrated and synthesized whole with "human relationship" as its nucleus.

1.6. FUNDAMENTAL PRINCIPLES FOR SOCIAL STUDIES COURSE

Following are some of the *basic principles for Social Studies*:

1. Social studies is an inter-disciplinary course. It draws its contents selectively from several other branches of knowledge and human experience.

2. It is the applied branch of Social Sciences. It is included in school curriculum so as to developing proper attitudes, sensibilities and skills in future citizens.
3. Its scope is ever growing, as the social process and problems are changing from time to time. Hence its content will have to be revised periodically.
4. Its approach in teaching is based on a pragmatic philosophy to serve the present requirements of a particular society and humanity and to help pupils to have social adjustment in their future lives, in their country and world.
5. Its field covers the study of communities at all levels - local, regional, national and international, with emphasis on man and his social environment.
6. It lays more emphasis on the contemporary human life and its problems as compared to that on the past history of man.
7. Its contents are useful as a media for general education at school level, before collegiate specialization starts so that pupils can learn them with sufficient case and interest.

1.7. RELATIONSHIP OF SOCIAL STUDIES TO OTHER SUBJECTS OF THE SCHOOL CURRICULUM

Social Studies units provide situations wherein the school children can use related learnings in a functional setting. This subject can provide a natural setting for the application and use of knowledge and basic skills in solving human problems. So it may rightly be used as a means of integrating various school activities and experiences.

Relationship between Physical Science and Social Studies

There exists a very close relationship between physical science and social studies. The units dealing with various human needs such as food, clothing, shelter, weather, transport and communications are dealt with in both social studies and physical sciences. The recent advances in science and technology has revolutionised the human life the world over and has brought man and man and nation and nation closer to each other. It has helped man to conquer space and time.

While teaching social studies we tell our students about the conditions needed to grow various types of plants and trees which are useful to man in one way or the other. The topics in social studies also deals with health and hygiene, cleanliness and sanitation etc. Similarly various topics of mathematics, biology, astronomy etc., are also included in social studies curricula. The life and work of great scientists of the world forms an essential part of the studies in social studies.

In these the teacher of social studies is required to trace the history of science and he is expected to work very closely with science master. Any advance in science and technology has always to be taken note of as it is going to affect social relations to a great extent. The present day civilisation has been built up on such scientific advances. Thus the two, i.e., physical sciences and social studies are closely related to each other.

Relationship between Language and Social Studies

Language is the media of communication between the teacher and the taught. In any system of education and for teaching of any subject language is of fundamental importance. Reading and writing and social studies are closely related. The child is expected to read a lot of printed material which is a vast source of social studies information. He is also required to express it either orally or in writing and it is only through such expressions that a child is evaluated by his teacher. During the social studies period the student is provided with enough of opportunities for discussing, speaking, debating, paper reading etc., in addition to providing the opportunity to do the written work. For all these activities a student has to depend on the knowledge of language and so the two are quite related to each other.

Relationship between Art and Social Studies

Various art activities are also closely related to Social Studies. In Social Studies, pupils are required to draw pictures, graphs, maps, diagrams, cartoons, time-lines, weather charts and many similar things. They are also required to prepare models of buildings, projects and dams and stage scenery for dramatic performances. Thus a large number of art and craft activities such as "Beautifying the school campus" and "Presenting a Mock Assembly or Panchayat" etc. can be taken up by pupils as an important part of Social Studies programme.

Relationship between Mathematics and Social Studies

Mathematics is also closely related to Social Studies as it provides speed and accuracy. Mathematical price lists, vouchers, cash memos and measurements provide practical experience to our pupils in money transactions, weights, time and measures. Similarly budgeting the expenditure within a given income, at subject, school, and family levels, helps in understanding the municipal, state and central government budgets. Then average rainfall and temperature of a place are calculated with mathematical calculations. Thus both the subjects can be correlated and associated on many occasions.

Thus, while teaching Social Studies, the pupils can be provided with opportunities for applying in a purposeful manner, many things that they have learnt in other areas of the curriculum.

1.8. SCOPE OF SOCIAL STUDIES

The scope of a subject defines the parameters of study of the subject such as the depth, comprehensiveness, variety etc.

Writing about the breadth of social studies John O. Michaels observes, "The breadth of Social Studies programme should provide for a variety of experiences so that the child's learning will be well-rounded and well-balanced. It should also be possible to draw upon other fields of learning so that significant problems can be considered in the light of their many ramifications; a narrow compartmentalized programme limits social learning."

In its comprehensiveness any Social Studies programme should meet the needs of individuals as also the needs of society and must be related to the problems and situations of daily life. Experience has shown that the majority of children learn most easily by dealing with concrete things and by adopting a course based on their own day-to-day experiences. This implies that the local environment should be the basis for acquainting children with the social environment. This will also ensure intelligibility and extension of experience rather than mere cramming.

As Social Studies programme has to be varied, it must draw such materials from all social sciences and even from natural sciences, as bears a direct relationship with the purposes for which this subject is taught.

(a) Vastness of Scope

The scope of social studies is very vast. It is as wide as the world and as long as the history of man. It is a study of human relationship and includes the following areas of relationships. Relationships between:

(i) People and people

(ii) People and institutions

(iii) People and Earth

(iv) People and Goods.

To understand these relationships it is essential that the student is provided with a basic knowledge of history, geography, economics, civics etc. Moreover all these subjects commonly referred to as social sciences should be synthesized into a compact whole by blending them together. It helps to remove limitations of each subject.

(b) Functional Study of Natural Sciences and Fine Arts

The social science and natural sciences are different areas of study but they are quite interdependent on each other. To illustrate the point we just cite the example of recent advances in science and technology that have totally revolutionised the social life in all parts of the world. The vision of man now goes far beyond his family, neighbourhood, nation etc. and expanded the area of human relationship to international level. The knowledge of physics, chemistry, botany, zoology, physiology etc. all are required in the study of social studies e.g. we have to teach in social studies how chemistry has helped in eradicating various diseases from the world. We have also to teach in social studies about the past experiences of human beings with diseases and the various researches and discoveries that helped to eradicate these diseases.

Then the functional study of fine arts such as drawing, constructing, painting, music, dance and dramatization, is also included in the curriculum of Social Studies. These arts provide the content that is needed for a better understanding of people and the world. The functional approach means that whatever factual material is obtained from various fields, must have immediate relationship to the needs and interests of children. Social Studies should mean something *happening* to pupils and teachers and not merely something *studied* by them.

(c) A Study of Current Affairs

Current affairs are those events that deal with our present problems and issues. Every current affair finds its background in the past. So it provides a great source of both historical and geographical learning.

A study of current affairs is helpful in weaving our present with our past and in this way help in complete learning. Current affairs are of great value as they represent an extension and exemplification of the different topics of curriculum of social studies.

(d) International Understanding

One of the objectives of any educational programmes is the promotion of international understanding. We are living in an atmosphere of fear and insecurity and the existing order is of full selfishness, injustice and exploitation. To overcome these social evils and to re-establish faith in basic human goodness we must emphasize on these values. The Indian children must learn "Brotherhood of mankind" and for this he should be made familiar with his personal needs, the needs of society as also the various problems that arise in modern day society by living together.

(e) Practical Study of Different Resources

In social studies curriculum we must include such new elements like character education, civil rights, cooperatives, social behaviour, inter-cultural relations and planning etc. It would be better to undertake excursions and visits to different towns and places of historical, economical, cultural, geographical, scientific and educational importance. The students of social studies should be given a good exposure to library and community resources, social service activities etc.

The study of social studies includes the history of mankind which goes millions of years prior to recorded history.

Above discussion make it abundantly clear that the scope of social studies is limitless and that it derives its subject-matter from all social sciences and related disciplines as also from literature, fine arts, physical sciences, religion etc. Thus it provides a wide range of materials. However, from it we must not conclude that its scope is limitless that has no ends. To limit its scope we have to keep in mind that it provides only the *functional* knowledge from various subjects leaving aside that material which has no bearing on human relationships. It thus contains only simple and reorganised piece of information from various subjects that is of practical importance in every day life of the child. In social studies we follow the principle of '*maximum essential.*'

REVISION QUESTIONS

1. Discuss the relationship of social studies with other school subjects.
2. Write a brief note on the scope of social studies and assess the importance of social studies in school curriculum.
3. Discuss the nature and scope of teaching social studies as a composite and integrated subject of school curriculum.
4. Clearly bring out the difference between social sciences and social studies.
5. Justify the place of social studies in school curriculum.
6. "The subject of social studies is all embracing in the sense that it concerns and teaches all aspects of human life." Discuss.
7. Do you prefer a composite course of social studies to the teaching of history, geography and civics as separate subjects? Give reasons with suitable examples in support of your answer.

2

Need and Importance of Social Studies

2.1. INTRODUCTION

Any society takes care of its young through the home and the school. It is through its schools, that a society prepares its future citizens. In a developing society like ours this responsibility of the school is greater, because the school should not only transmit, from one generation to the next, our tradition and culture, but help in the process of modernisation. For discharging this responsibility, the school depends, among other things, heavily on the teaching of social studies, the central concern of which is to understand the relationship between man and his society.

A study of social studies helps us to develop a broad, rational, national and secular outlook. The Secondary Education Commission 1952-53 has observved, "The education system must make its contribution to the development of habits, attitudes and qualities of character, which will enable its citizens to bear worthily the responsibilities of democratic citizenships and to counteract all those fissiparous tendencies which hinder the emergence of a broad national and secular outlook."

2.2. NEED AND IMPORTANCE OF SOCIAL STUDIES

In the olden days the child learnt about interpersonal relationship of his group at his home where he was provided with rich activities to know about the relationship that existed between him and his environments. All these experiences were enough to provide him with the social education that he required. With advances in science and technology we find more of individual life and the joint family system has almost disappeared. The child is thus deprived of social education at home. This function of providing the social education is now expected to be performed by schools. To provide such a social education school curriculum must include material that would acquaint the child with the best of the traditions in society that existed in the past. This material should also enable the child to solve his every day problems of living and should also prepare him to deal intelligently his future problems. All this can be achieved by adopting a unified course of social studies.

We should provide the young child with the maximum of information about the social and environmental realities of the past. Previously the human relationships were taught under separate subjects such as history, geography, economics, etc. and each subject was concerned with a particular type of relationship. These subjects were overcrowded with various details which have become irrelevant and burdensome in the present day society. Due to these drawbacks the social studies emerged as a new field of studies. In the words of Dr. Radha Krishnan, the great philospher and statesman, ''Let us remember the past, be alive to present and create the future with courage in our hearts and faith in ourselves.''

At present our aim is to ensure complete national integration and establish a truly democratic, socialist society. It is a gigantic task and we have to tackle such a difficult problem. We have a glorious past, with remarkable tradition of peace, tolerance and assimilation. The pancea for all our problems lies in recapturing the ancient spirit. We are required to take living fire from the past and constantly recreate traditions. A revolution in thought and outlook is a must to achieve some thing new, i.e., democratic nationalism. It can be achieved through an integrated course of social studies in which an attempt is made to interpret the past in the context off present day situations.

With our Independence in 1947, we started with the task of building a socialistic, democratic society. In such a society we expect equal opportunity of work to success for even the humblest individual alongwith the most powerful and influential. It all is possible only in a welfare state. To achieve this our educational system is expected to concentrate on providing the future citizens with certain attitudes and skills. The school should produce such citizens who are well-informed and discriminating patriots and democrats, without caste, class and linguistic bias. This can be achieved to a great extent by introducing social studies in our school curriculum.

2.3. SOCIAL STUDIES AS A CORE SUBJECT

To understand the utility of a subject in school curriculum it is essential for us to know the function of education and the content of education. It is on the basis of such a knowledge that we will be able to justify the inclusion of any subject in our school curriculum.

In a democratic country every individual is expected to live a democratic life, with satisfaction to himself and with profit to his society. All this can be achieved only through education. One of the important functions of education therefore is " Preparation for life." The education should enable a child to live as self-sufficient, useful and healthy individual. It should also enable him to live as a home member, a worker and a citizen. To achieve all this, a *functional content of education* is essential. Such a content will not only create a sense of values in life, it will also formulate desirable patterns of attitudes and behaviour. It will also, create in child, a love of life and confidence in mankind.

The basic content of Social Studies is drawn from different subjects such as history, geography, civics, economics, etc. and it comprises of material on "**Man and his Environment.**" It would be better if such a course content is taught as a compulsory subject upto secondary school stage of education which might be the final stage of education for a majority of the children. The following are some of the reasons to teach Social Studies as a core subject upto secondary school stage of education.

1. Psychological Reason

Psychologists believe that man is a creation of environment and his personality is best developed in that environment. Any human being is always curious to know more and more about his environment so as to interpret it correctly. He is always willing to respond to his environment. In the olden days the inter personal relationship was established by direct participation of men in the environment but these days, due to absence of joint family system, even this has to be taught in schools. From amongst different school subjects it is only the Social Studies where a child can be taught about his relationship with his environment. It is in this context that the teaching of social studies as a core subject in our schools assumes importance.

Presently an effort is made to deal with all our problems in a psychological way and one is made to believe that he is to live alongwith others. A child needs a specific type of behaviour to deal with people, not only to interact but also to understand the interaction of others. To achieve all this the Social Studies must be given its due place in school curriculum. In Social Studies the subject starts with concrete things and it "deals with the substance of life, for life and assimilated through living."

2. Educational Reasons

The three basic aims of education are:

(i) Material

(ii) Cultural and

(iii) Social.

Material aim of education is that the child should be able to earn his livelihood and thus education should prepare a child for some vocation. It is also referred to as the *utilitarian* aim of education.

The education should bring about a complete and harmonious development of the child's personality and it includes the development of all capacities of an individual. It is the *cultural* aim of education.

Since the child has to be a member of the society so we must keep **social** aim of education in mind. In the present day democratic society each one of us is expected to participate in the decision-making process on all events having national or even international importance. It, therefore, becomes quite essential that education make a real contribution towards the development of the child to understand his own nature, the nature of his physical and social environment and also about his place in this environment. The education should make the child more social minded, truthful, honest, loyal, tolerant, and cooperative. To achieve all this a great effort and a total overhaul of the system of education is required. The major thrust should be to make necessary changes in the material content of education and the methods of teaching. The teacher should make full use of various educational aids available to him such as cinema, wireless, audio-visual aids etc. He should try to make use of newly developed teaching methods such as *project method, activity method* etc. To achieve maximum benefit from these it should be set in an integrated course of study and this is what we try to achieve in Social Studies.

3. Sociological Reasons

As made clear in the previous discussion the aim of education is to inculcate in child the social awareness. This aim of education can be fulfilled to a large extent by the study of Social Studies. In Social Studies the child is taught, how the society has come to its present form from its past days. Various past achievements of society and their effect on the present are also taught to the child. He is also provided the necessary knowledge about various changes in physical and social environment that has taken place during this transition of society from past to present. It is expected that the knowledge about all these things will produce well adjusted citizens who will be prepared to solve their problems. It thus clearly establishes the reason for teaching of Social Studies as a compulsory subject upto the secondary school stage of education.

4. Practical Reasons

It has been argued that a child who has studied Social Studies inculcates such ideals and attitudes which make him a more successful and practical man. These are the basic requirements of any adult citizen of the day. Thus the Social Studies must be taught as a compulsory subject at the school stage.

From the above discussion we can easily conclude that the inclusion of Social Studies as a compulsory subject in our schools will enable the young generation to adjust itself to the changing world and will help in producing selfreliant and enlightened citizens for our newly born democracy.

REVISION QUESTIONS

1. Discuss the importance of Social Studies as a compulsory school subject.
2. Discuss in brief the need and importance of Social Studies as a school subject.
3. Discuss the various reasons that support the inclusion of Social Studies as a core subject in our school curriculum.
4. Justify the place of Social Studies in Secondary School curriculum.
5. Why has Social Studies been included as one of the core subjects in the curriculum upto secondary classes ?

3

Functions, Aims and Values of Teaching Social Studies

3.1. INTRODUCTION

For proper teaching of a subject it is essential to have a knowledge of aims and objectives of the subject. This is also true for the teaching of social studies. Various methods of teaching are then evolved according to these aims and objectives. For determining the aims of teaching any subject we have to take into consideration the utility and usefulness of that subject. We have material as well as spiritual aspects in our life. For a successful spiritual life it is essential that we have a well founded material life.

The aims and objectives of teaching various subjects are normally very similar and they are generally guided by economic and social considerations. The aims and objectives of teaching Social Studies include all the aims and objectives of education. Different writers have listed these aims and objectives in different ways. In case of social studies, it is said that, "The outstanding purpose of instructions in social studies is to produce citizens and to aid pupils in the formation of a higher type of social studies character."

3.2. FUNCTIONS OF SOCIAL STUDIES

The important functions of social studies are:

1. Social Experience

Social studies provides social experiences to our pupils. Though child has varied social experiences with his parents, relations, neighbours, relatives, friends etc. before he joins the school but in school he gains new and varied experiences as he interacts with his classmates, teachers and others. In his classes he is also taught about family, religion, nation etc. It also provides him with social experiences.

2. Social Skills

To make his social experiences meaningful he is also provided with the skills and techniques to apply his experiences into practical life. Social skills are as important as the skills of reading, writing etc. The social skills help an individual in building up a healthy, vigorous and dynamic society. The social skills include respect and consideration for others, toleration of differences, adjustment of opposition, accommodation and compromises. Social studies contributes to provide for all these skills either directly or indirectly.

3. Social Knowledge

In addition to providing social experiences and social skills a study of social studies also provides a lot of information regarding man relationships. The child acquires this knowledge in various ways such as through reading, through pictures etc. This knowledge helps the child to know the correct facts and helps him to make correct interpretations, judgements and generalisations.

4. Social Standards

Every society has a certain code of social standards for its members. These generally include that the individual member of the society should speak the truth, obey the law, perform his duties and maintain a desirable behaviour. Any group is not expected to oppress individual members. Similar behaviour is expected from other social institutions such as church, school etc. In social studies the student is familiarised with all such social standards that the society has evolved during its development. It provides the child with education for character, and behaviour and also for the formation of attitudes, ideals and standards.

5. Social Problems

One of the functions of the teaching of social studies is to make the child realise that society has failed to solve certain problems.

This will enable the child to participate in social progress. In social Studies there are unlimited opportunities for such problems that society has failed to solve.

6. Social Changes

Recent advances in science and technology has brought about many a changes in our socialset up. These advances have only very changed the physical environment but also have brought about tremendous changes in social environment. They have changed the social order at a very fast rate. Actually the change has become our constant companion. To be able to cope with these changes and to act intelligently the child should be made to understand this changing nature of the present world and its dynamic content. This function is performed by an integrated course of social studies.

From the above discussion the different functions of social studies become quite clear and it also helps to clarify the nature of social studies. It also identifies the social purpose that is expected to be served by teaching of social studies in schools.

3.3. AIMS OF TEACHING OF SOCIAL STUDIES

Aims are broad general statements that communicate long range purposes or intentions. A very general aim can be broken down into different kinds of objectives. Objectives are more precise statements of purpose. The aims and objectives cannot remain the same in all times and under all circumstances. The teacher should utilize these aims and objectives in such a way that he may produce ideal citizens of the country. Some important aims of teaching social studies are given below:

1. To Enrich and Develop the Lives of Pupils within their Environment

To achieve it the child be provided with the knowledge about how the environment came into being, what is the influence of environment on an individual and on the community. The pupils should be able to appreciate the inter-relationship of the elements of their environments through the integrated subject-matter from diffferent subjects such as history, geography, civics, sociology etc. They should also be told about the past and present struggles of mankind and encouraged to contribute in the future progress of society. They must be thoroughly acquainted with the development of past institutions like state, church and business concerns etc. and also the changes that have taken place in their character with the changing times.

2. Acquisition of Knowledge and Understanding

Acquisition of definite amount of knowledge is essential for good citizenship. This contributes directly to social progress because exact knowledge is essential for clear thinking and sound judgement. Knowledge also satisfies the natural curiosity of pupils, quickens their imagination and helps them in building up individual interests. Without clear thinking and critical judgement, many problems of modern civilization cannot be solved. Knowledge is also the basis of sympathy and understanding which are so essential for intercourse and social solidarity. Definite knowledge of Social Studies promotes understanding of all history and all human experience as a process of change and development. It also makes clear to pupils that social changes are inevitable as a result to scientific advancement and that individualism should give place to collectivism.

Some of the important characteristics of good citizen are as follows:

A good citizen

(i) Believes in equality of opportunity for all people.

(ii) Values, respects and defends basic human rights and privileges guaranteed by our constitution.

(iii) Respects and upholds the law and its various agencies.

(iv) Understands and accepts the democratic principles.

(v) Puts the general welfare above his own welfare.

(vi) Exercises his right of vote freely.

(vii) Accepts his civic responsibility and discharges them to the best of his capability.

(viii) Realises the necessary connection of education with democracy.

(ix) Assumes a personal responsibility for the wise use of natural resources.

(x) Understands cultures and ways of life other than his own.

(xi) Supports all efforts to prevent war, but is always ready to defend his country against tyranny and aggression.

(xii) Cultivates qualities of character and personality that have a high value in his culture.

(xiii) Recognises taxes as payment for community services and pays them promptly.

(xiv) In a responsible family member and assumes his full responsibility for maintaining the civic standards of his neighbourhood and community.

(xv) Is guided by the idea of "Live and Let Live."

Writing about citizenship H.H. Horne observes, "Citizenship is a man's place in the States. As the state is one of the permanent institutions of society and as man must ever live in organised relation with his fellows citizenship cannot be omitted from the constituency of the educational ideal."

3. Training in Desirable Patterns of Conduct

In the olden days home and church played an important role in the educational process of children. But now both home and church have ceased to play their important role in the development of character and behaviour of children to the desired extent. Now the entire burden of training children in the right type of behaviour and conduct is to be borne by the school. It is therefore, the duty of the school to develop desirable patterns of conduct among children and thus help in the building up of character so as to produce good citizens. The Social Studies teacher is in a position to inculcate all this by virtue of the subject-matter that he teaches and the method that he follows.

4. Development of Right Attitudes

Development of right attitudes is also one of the major aims of teaching Social Studies. Desirable attitudes are essential because they are extremely significant factors of behaviour. They are based on an appreciation of things which are worth-while in life. Attitudes depend upon intellectual and emotional factors. Scientific attitudes is intellectual because in it judgements are based on facts, unaffected by personal feelings but emotional attitudes depend to a large extent on individuals. It is expected from the teacher that he will help his pupils in building up the right attitudes. In order to obtain good results the teacher must show self-control, patience, sympathy and self-respect.

5. Strengthening National and International Integration

In a vast country like India, a member of fissiparous tendencies are likely to exist and such tendencies may threaten the unity of country. This is a serious problem. A proper teaching of social studies can help to create a sound base for the continued oneness and unity of country.

With the development of science and technology, the barriers of time are space and crumbling down. It is not far off, when the whole world will become a single unit. Any citizen of a country will then not be able to keep himself away from the ways of other countries. A man can be a real citizen of his country only when he possesses an international outlook. Such an outlook will help him to acquire the attitude of 'Co-existence' or the principle of 'Live and Let Live'.

All this will create in our students a realization of interdependency of man and man and nation and nation. It will also help them understand each others problems and their solutions.

6. Socialization of Pupils

Socialization will awaken in pupils a sense of role which will help to develop in them confidence, courage and happiness. It will also develop individual and social virtues of initiative, truthfulness, righteousness, constructive thinking, critical judgement, justice, tolerance, cooperation, fellow feeling, sacrifice etc.

A list of 16 commonly accepted aims of teaching Social Studies in USA given by R.C.A. Edwin is as follows:

I. To Impart Knowledge and Understanding, i.e.

1. To make the child understand his natural environment so as to enable him to adjust better in his physical, social and cultural environment.

2. To acquire and understand social concepts of family, community, state and nation.
3. To acquire information about the world around him and thus broaden his field of interests.
4. To develop an appreciation of social heritage.
5. To make him know the progress of society from the primitive to the advanced and that of the culture, pattern and contemporary actions and the results of inter-weaving of history, environment and character.
6. To acquaint the child about man, his ways of living, his significant achievements and his institutions and the problems that he faces today.
7. To help the child to understand how far geographical conditions influenced in moulding growth of society in different parts of world.
8. To help the child to learn about vocational activities and opportunities.

II. To Develop Desirable Attitudes, i.e.

9. To assume social and civic responsibility and thus making the child an actively participating and enlightened citizen.
10. To act in accordance with democratic principles and values.
11. To develop attitudes of personal responsibility, civic and world mindedness, emotional maturity, intellectual integrity, aesthetic appreciation and sound judgement.

III. To Give Training in Desirable Patterns of Conduct, i.e.

12. To inculcate the habits of patriotism, courage, co-operation and toleration.
13. To enable the child to appreciate the view-points of others and to make his own contribution.

IV. To Initiate and Improve Basic Skills, i.e.

14. To help the child to develop such skills as are necessary for effective participation in social life.
15. To develop critical and scientific thinking and give sense of time.

16. To inculcate the following social studies skills:
    (a) to interpret printed, pictured and charted material;
    (b) to place people, events and institutions in time, space and importance;
    (c) to use words of social and economic significance correctly;
    (d) to understand and interpret significant dates and to compare contrast, summarize, generalize and criticize them.

If social studies is taught with these aims then we will be able to produce good and useful citizens and an ideal society. For fulfilment of these aims systematic plans have to be formulated. In any such plan teacher occupies the central place because he is the person to carry most of the burden and is required to work in the field to realise these aims.

3.4. VALUES OF TEACHING SOCIAL STUDIES

Before we discuss the values of teaching social studies let us make clear the difference between aims and values.

Aims are conscious purposes and goals whereas **values** are outcomes or results achieved after teaching according to those aims.

Thus **aims** are **desired goals** whereas values are **expected outcomes.**

Aims are based on **philosophy** whereas **values** are based on **reality.**

Outcomes are more important as they deal with actual values which are achieved through instructions after deciding definite aims or objectives.

By teaching of social studies properly in accordance with the aims already described, it is expected to give the following outcomes:

1. Social Learning

In the olden times knowledge was provided in the form of separate subjects like history, geography, civics etc., because much of the social learning was provided to the child at his home which used to be the real centre of social learning and provided all the necessary background. Since the home nowadays does not provide any such environment for most of our children so the need for an integrated course of social studies was felt. This subject will give the child social education and social awareness will help to refrain the child from anti-social influences. It will also help to build up the social understanding of the child.

2. Knowledge with Experience

It is not enough to provide the child with bookish knowledge as it will give the child an idea that anything written in the book is correct and so he will develop a blind faith in anything that appears in prints. In social studies an attempt is made to create situations that provide the child a chance to learn by doing and by experiencing. From these experiences it becomes clear to the child that even the teachers and books may always be not correct. They also understand that learning is a continuous process and he also can share it.

3. Competence in Tackling Problems

A child who is overburdened with factual knowledge may gain an impression that for each problem there is a readymade solution available in books. However, when a child is taught social studies by project method or problem method he has to tackle the problem in his own way and this leads to self-reliance which leads to sense of responsibility. By completing the project himself the child begins to feel that he can do things himself. It creates enough confidence in the child to face situations boldly and to solve successfully the problem in hand.

4. Training in Co-operation

Co-operation in school work is quite rare among school children. They are generally found struggling for personal attainment and for gaining more marks than their fellows. Co-operation in school is shown only in the playing fields or in some other co-curricular activities. The same thing is observed in adult life. Everyone adopts individualistic attitude with his fellows in his daily life. Such an attitude is not desirable these days. Because under changed circumstances, we need work-relationships and co-operation, more than anything else, for the very existence and survival of our nation.

No doubt, a certain amount of school work must also be individualistic. We have to look to special aptitudes, natural endowments and abilities of our pupils and give them opportunities for individual advancement. But Social Studies will provide "the necessary corrective for too much indivualism" by creating situations for co-operative work inside the class-room.

5. Help for the Slow and the Backward

Social studies is quite helpful for the slow, dull and backward children. Since they fail to master successfully the narrow fields of factual knowledge provided by history, geography, civics etc., as separate subjects so they suffer constant discouragements at the hands of their teachers as also from their comparatively bright fellow students Such discouragement generally leads to abnormalities of children. Social studies, however, provides ample opportunities to each child for making his or her useful contribution even if he or she is comparatively less intellectual.

6. Adjustability and Flexibility

Because of scientific inventions and technical advances of the last seventy years, the human life has changed to a great extent. These rapid changes can foretell what lies in the future. So while educating the child, we must keep an eye on the shape of things to come at least 25-30 years after. This will help the child in developing a flexible outlook and will enable him to adjust himself to the changes that will take place in his adult life. This can be achieved through a unified course of social studies that will teach children that "life is a continual process of growth." It will also tell him how to participate intelligently in that process and how to adjust himself properly to changing environments.

7. Skill in Selection

The traditional curriculum fails to tell the young child that successful living is a process of wise selection. Civilization is becoming more and more complex and so the ability to select wisely from the available variety, has become exceedingly necessary though it is quite difficult. It is social studies that provides constant practice in wise selection, both for teachers and pupils. The course itself, ''calls for decisions about the topics to be taken up for detailed discussion, the topics to be taken up superficially and the topics to be omitted from the syllabi. In Social Studies the child gets sufficient opportunities to find out what has for them of immediate relevance and the value. It also helps them in making a better choice of profession for themselves.

8. Development of the Power of Thinking and Reasoning

The subject-matter of social studies that is drawn from different subjects such as history, geography, civics etc., aims to provide our young children, who are the future citizens, some true understanding of the mankind through the ages. He is told about the glorious past of man and the way he learnt to control his environment. He is told about different institutions that existed in the past society and how they changed according to the needs of the times. All this factual knowledge helps the child in developing his power of thinking and reasoning.

This power of thinking and reasoning helps the child information of judgements and ultimately to solution of problems. Since in a democratic society each individual is expected to participate in deciding matter of national or even international importance so this knowledge of social studies is quite helpful to the child to participate effectively in solving the problems that he faces.

9. A Sense of Personal Role

You must have observed many persons who prefer to remain aloof and are self-centred. Such persons are those who have become desocialised. Such persons fail to grasp the simple fact that it is possible for them to lead a better and happier lives by social cooperation. Social studies will not only teach them about the organisation of social structure, but it will also provide them some experience of cooperative work. The teaching of social studies will awaken in young students a consciousness of social role that is so essential for personal and social advancement.

From the preceding discussion we conclude that most of the appropriate objectives of teaching social studies, as given by R.C.A. Edwin for American society, are quite relevant to Indian conditions. India has accepted democracy both as a form of government and as a way of life.

REVISION QUESTIONS

1. Make out a clear distinction between aims and values.
2. Discuss in brief the values of teaching of Social Studies.
3. Give a brief description of important functions of Social Studies.
4. Discuss the importance of aims and objectives for teaching of any subject.
5. Give an outline of the various values of teaching of Social Studies.

4

The Contents of Social Studies

4.1. INTRODUCTION

'Curriculum' may be defined as the 'social environment in motion.' It is the sum total of all the activities and experiences provided by the school to the learners for achieving the desired objectives. The courses of studies are merely a suggestion for curriculum activities and procedures, a guide for teaching to follow.

Curriculum is the pivot and hub around which all activities in school revolve. Curriculum in Social Studies is the part of the school curriculum which includes the subject-matter and experiences that is intended to acquire an understanding of human relations, provide knowledge of basic principles and values of society, inculcate right attitudes, develop appropriate skills, teach tolerance, cultivate a forward outlook, impart mental training, help resolve contemporary, individual and social problems, foster national feelings and develop international understanding.

Edgar Bruce Wesley has rightly remarked, "The curriculum is an educational instrument, planned and used by the school to effect its purposes."

According to Payne, "curriculum consists of all the situations that school may select and consciously organise for the purpose of developing the personality of its pupils and for making behaviour changes in them."

It is, in fact, a means of which the child adjusts himself to his environment. The knowledge of the fact that experience is the best teacher gives a new approach to curriculum. Thus both content and activity are kept in view while framing curriculum in social studies.

4.2. NEED FOR THE PLANNING OF CURRICULUM

The word *'curriculum'* is derived from the Latin word *'curresve'* which means to run. So curriculum is a course of path on which one runs to reach a goal. Thus curriculum includes the subject-matter and all learning experiences arranged by the school for a particular subject.

The needs of life go on changing so is education, so we cannot go on with a static curriculum. The content has to be selected according to the changing needs of the society in general and subject-matter in particular. The curriculum has to be planned and organised in a scientific manner keeping in view the psychological requirements of the students. If the curriculum is properly organised, it enables the students to know the subject-matter which they have to study. On the other hand, it also makes clear to the teacher, the material that they have to teach to the students. It also provides the same facility to the examiner.

The contents of social studies is only a framework of suggested topics suited to different ages and stages. These topics may be selected and developed according to the needs and abilities of the pupils in different grades. Actually, "Selecting, grading and organising the contents of the curriculum are the tasks of the teacher," who knows the limitations as well as the capacities of his students. The Social Studies teacher therefore must possess a flexible mind, a nature sense of values, an awareness of essentials and sufficient creative imagination" to be able to dispense with this task successfully.

4.3 IMPORTANCE OF THE CURRICULUM

Curriculum is one of the most important items in the educative process. It is useless to talk of **how** or **when** to teach without first deciding **what** to teach. The curriculum, in fact, is the fundamental problem which determines the "warp and woof" of the process education. **What** to do and **how** to do, are the very essence of curriculum. Curriculum is a medium through which the pupils make an effort to achieve the objectives of education. In addition to it "curriculum acts as a pivot in organising educational effort on some manageable basis and is undoubtedly the heart of the school and all that goes with it." The school must provide knowledge and experience to its pupils if it wishes to produce really useful members for our democratic society. These ends can only be met by a well-planned curriculum in every subject.

4.4. CONSTRUCTION OF CURRICULUM

The following two stages are important in the construction of curriculum:

(i) Selection of the curriculum, and

(ii) Organisation of curriculum material.

(i) Principles of Selection of the Curriculum

Tradition is not going to be our guiding principle in the selection and arrangement of the subject-matter. It is not possible or advisable to carry out the selection of a curriculum in a haphazard manner. Curriculum has to be properly planned and to be based on certain principles. These principles will be discussed now.

Principles of the Selection of Curriculum or Subject-matter

Though the organisation of various information and subject-material is a difficult task, yet educationists have tried to lay down certain principles, on the basis of which, the subject-material or the content material of civics may be organised. Some of these are as follows:

(a) Principle of Utility (or use)

Knowledge for the sake of knowledge is a good aim but in the existing circumstance it is not a successful aim. At present we have to keep in mind the utilitarian aspect of every subject-matter. If the subject-matter is not of any use the students will not feel interested in it for a long time. Thus the curriculum material should include only those topics which are useful for a particular grade in many ways. Firstly, an attempt be made to include those topics which are useful in day-to-day life. The curriculum material of the subject should have the following ingredients in it.

(i) It should be useful in every day life.

(ii) It should be useful in the study of other subjects.

(iii) It should have some vocational utility.

(iv) It should enable students to understand and appreciate the role played by civics in the development of civilization and other branches of knowledge.

(b) Principle of Disciplinary Value

Teaching of social studies disciplines the mind. Previously this was the sole criterion to select the subject-matter. This brought into syllabus much useless material. The students used to study certain puzzles and riddles which had no practical utility. For disciplining the mind, one topic is as good as another. Unless and until it topic has some other values, it should not be included in the curriculum simply for its disciplinary value. Real useful problems train the mind better than unreal formal problems. When the students can get both useful knowledge and mental training from the same set of facts, it is not wise to make pupils learn one set of facts for mental exercise and another for the acquisition of knowledge. In the words of Thorndike, "Teach nothing merely because of its disciplinary value but teach everything so as to get, what disciplinary value it does have."

(c) Principle of Cultural Value

Social studies has played an important role in the advancement of culture and civilisation. There may be certain ideas that were pursued by the students of social studies which may not be of any use now. But there are certain ideas and facts of civics that form an integral part of modern culture and society. Such facts or ideas should be included in the curriculum. Their study will be a source of inspiration to the students.

(d) Principle of Preparatory Value

The material of the curriculum should be so selected that it should be preparatory as well as terminus. On the one hand, it should train the students for life and on the other it should also prepare them for higher education. The content should include the topics which prepare the child (i) for university education, (ii) for life. Only a small percentage of the students go up to the university stage and for most of them school is a terminal stage. Hence, the requirements of college course need not dominate the school curriculum. After every stage of education some students enter life while others go into for higher education. The curriculum should be such as to be able to provide satisfactory education to both these categories of students.

(e) Principle of Child Centredness

Social studies is a very vast subject so it becomes difficult to make a selection of the things which are useful to the students. For taking a decision about usefulness of the content material we should always keep in mind the child for whom it is meant. Do not forget that curriculum is for child and the child is not for the curriculum. While making a selection of useful topics for inclusion in curriculum childs' interests, abilities, age levels, etc., should be kept in mind. The duration of the course should also be given due consideration while making the selection of topics for inclusion in the curriculum. An attempt be made to provide in the curriculum topics for various categories of students.

(f) Principle of Community Centredness

Since every child has to live in and for the community, it would be desirable that he is able to live well in society. In the curriculum of Social Studies all such topics be included which cater to the needs of the society. Thus an attempt be made to shape the curriculum according to the needs of the society.

(g) Principle of Flexibility

The aim of education as also the aims of teaching a subject go on changing because they depend on the needs of ever changing society. The developments in the subject also necessitate a change in curriculum. Thus it is not possible for us to follow any rigid curriculum forever. The curriculum has to be modified and reviewed quite frequently so as to shape it according to the latest developments of the subject. It is essential if we have to keep pace with the modern world. In this regards the views be sought from subject specialists.

(h) Principle of Activity

Educationists are of the views that 4 H's should find a place in the curriculum. In other words, it means that the content material should be based on these 4 H's. These H's are nothing but Health,

Head, Hands and Heart. It means that a co-ordination should be established between the hands and the mind. Such a co-ordination would enable the children to act intelligently. Such activities should be given place in the curriculum that may lead to the activity of the children. Child is by nature active. His path of activity and agility should not be beset with difficulties. If it is beset with difficulties his progress will be retarded. The organisation and selection of the subject-material of Social Studies should be based on activity. Such events, instances and topics of Social Studies should be included in the curriculum that lead to the activity in the child. The curriculum should also be so organised that it may bring about activity in the children.

(i) Principle of Utility

This is a world of selectivity. We follow the principle of pick choose in regard to subject material and activity. We take to activities and materials that are useful for our life and discard those that do not seem to be useful. Selection of that subject-material of Social Studies shall be useful which fulfills our educational needs.

Whitehead has classified the educational life into three parts or stages— (1) Romance, (2) Precision, and (3) Generalisation.

Precision is nothing but utility. Selection of the subject-material should be based on precision and utility. Material that is not precise and useful should not find a place in the teaching of Social Studies. By and by, with the development of various mental powers, the child is able to discriminate between useful and useless. He welcomes what is useful and discards what is not useful. If the content material of teaching is not based on the principle of utility, it shall not attract the students towards the study.

(j) Principle of Formality and Cultural Heritage

Every individual is proud of his or her cultural heritage. This is very true of India. We try to preserve the culture handed over to us by our forefathers. Alongwith it we also try to enrich it. This can be done if we include in the curriculum of teaching of Social Studies, the subject-material that helps preservation of culture and its enrichment. This is possible only if the subject-matter is selected on the basis of the principle of formality.

(k) Principle of Interest

In the modern education, interests, aptitude and other mental faculties play a vital role. Attempt is made to base the entire education in the interest of the children. In the teaching of Social Studies such subject-material should be selected which is of interest to the students. Selection will not be sufficient. It should be so organised that it is interesting to the educands. If the content material is not based on interest, children shall not feel inclined to study it. The whole education today is child-centred. It is, therefore, all the more necessary, to organise the subject-material of the Social Studies, with an eye on the interest of the child. In other words, the selection and organisation of the subject-material should be according to nature of the child.

(l) Principle of Selectivity

We cannot have each and everything in the curriculum. We have to follow the principle of pick and choose. Those things that are helpful for the betterment of the society and bring about the preservation of the social values and cultural standards are given place in the curriculum. The content material should be so organised that it may help the students to understand social and political problems. The material should be in accordance with the intelligence and mental power of the students.

(m) Principle of Concentric Growth

This principle indicates that we should proceed 'from known to unknown' and 'from concrete to abstract'. First of all, those facts should be presented before the child that are already known to him. Then facts unknown to him should be presented before him and they should be connected with the known facts. This means that while teaching Social Studies problems dealing with the local aspect of citizenship should be presented before the children. Then attempt should be made to present the national and international problems appertaining citizenship.

The child lives in the family. When he grows he comes in contact with his neighbourhood. Later on, he comes in contact with the town, the state, the country and the entire world. The knowledge and the teaching of Social Studies should begin with the knowledge of the family. First of all the teacher should try to present the citizenship before the child as it afffects his family. By and by, he should go on broadening this circle of knowledge. It is in the end that the citizenship of the world or world citizenship should come before the student.

(n) Teachers' Points of View

While framing or revising the curriculum, the views of teachers, who are the real workers, should also be sought. They know the levels of students and the thing which should be taught to the students. At present, the curriculum is imposed on the teachers and as such, they do not realise the significance of changes in the curriculum if any. The new trend expects participation and contribution from the teachers' side.

So we see while constructing curriculum for a grade, various considerations are to be kept in mind. Nothing should be included simply because of disciplinary value. Utility should provide the chief criterion of curriculum construction. Of course, the latest trends in the subject, the needs of community, the needs for students and above all, the views of the teachers should be given due weight in any scheme of curriculum construction.

View of J.W.A. Young in regard to Selection of the Subject-matter of Curriculum

According to Young, selection of subject-matter of curriculum should be guided by the following consideration (or principles).

1. To exhibit most clearly and to the best advantages the various political thoughts.
2. To help to a better understanding of society.
3. To bring out clearly the relationships between Social Studies and modern life and to show how Social Studies can help to solve various problems of life.
4. To allow the organisation of material into a homogeneous whole, meeting the demands of pedagogy.

4.5. ORGANISATION OF THE FACTS OR SUBJECT-MATTER

The second problem that we have to face in constructing curriculum or laying down the subject-material of teaching of Social Studies is the organisation of facts. The facts should be so organised that the students may acquire them and assimilate them thoroughly. For this various principles have been laid down. Some of these are as follows:

1. Psychological and Logical Arrangement

Logical arrangement leads to the rigorous treatment of the subject-matter which is based on logical reasoning whereas psychological arrangement is from the point of view of the students. It seems that both the approaches are different but these can be easily merged. The organisation can both be psychological and logical. All thinking is psychological. Psychological throws light on the power of understanding of students at a particular stage. We can be logical in various ways. Psychological should decide which logical approach will suit for a particular topic. Logic will help in maintaining proper sequence of topics, so we should organise the topics in such a way that we may follow Psychological and Logic at the same time. The happy combination of the two is always desirable.

Psychological organisation throws light on the use of a topic for the pupil from the academic as well as practical point of view. It takes into consideration the power of grasping and understanding of pupils in a particular age group. The order in which topics as to be taken up will largely depend on its findings. Similarly logic must be there. Psychological should decide what kind of logic is appropriate for the pupil of a certain age and what type will be suitable for the development of such logical thinking. Logic will help in maintaining the link and sequence of topics found useful and meaningful for the child.

Logical organisation of the subject-matter deals with the vigorous logical reasoning associated with the subjects.

2. Topical and Spiral Arrangement

Topical arrangement means that a topic should be finished entirely at one stage. It takes the topics as a unit. Spiral arrangement implies that a topic should be split up into different portions and these portions should be spread over different grades. Easier portions should be dealt with in the lower grades and the difficult portions should be gradually introduced in the next grade. The latter is definitely good arrangement. Topical arrangement requires that easy and diffficult portions of a topic should be dealt with at one stage which is unpsychological.

However simple or easy topics may be finished at one stage, while spiral arrangement is good, long grinding at all grades is undesirable. The selection of a particular approach will depend on the topic.

3. From Easy to Difficult

Organisation of the content material of the curriculum be done keeping in view the mental development and the capacities of the students. The easier topics should come first and difficult ones later on. However, we should bear in mind that what appears easy to the teacher, may not be easy to the students, so this is to seen from the point of view of the student. For this we have to keep in mind the mental level, capacities and age level of the students.

For any particular class only those topics be included in syllabus which are within the comprehension of the students.

4. Principle of Activity

The child likes activity and these days activity plays an important part in teaching of a subject-matter. Organisation of curriculum should not fail to suggest some practical work wherever it is possible. In lower classes those topics be included which put more emphasis on practical work. It helps in making clear various concepts in civics and thus help in developing a love for the subject.

Following activities be kept in mind while organising the subject-matter of curriculum:

(i) Personal and home activities.

(ii) Recreational activities.

(iii) Vocational activities.

(iv) Community, civic and social activities.

(v) National activities.

5. Principle of Correlation

While organising the content in Social Studies the principle of correlation should always be given due weightage. Correlation may be of different varieties. The following types of correlation must be kept in mind while organising curriculum in Social Studies:

(i) Correlation of Social Studies with the problems of every day life.

(ii) Correlation of Social Studies with other subjects.

(iii) Correlation between different branches of social sciences.

(iv) Correlation with craft or work experience.

For correlating subject-matter we must know the following:

(i) Day-to-day life activities of the students.

(ii) The nature of topics included in other subjects at the same stage.

(iii) The sequence of topics of the same branch of the subject.

(iv) The nature of work experience or project undertaken by the students.

6. Scope of Individual Teaching

Psychology shows that no two children are like. There are individual differences in students. The same type of rigid syllabus may not suit all the students. There may be ability grouping of students, i.e., the students of almost the same intelligence and achievement may be but in one group. Accordingly there should be grouping of topics in the curriculum. There should be different assignments for bright and dull students.

The most prevalent view at present is that the requirements of the groups as a whole should have priority over individual requirements. However, educationists differ in this regard and some of them emphasise that the subject-matter of the curriculum should be so arranged that the difference in the abilities of students are not neglected.

7. Voice of the Teacher

The teacher must have definite say in the selection and organisation of the curriculum in civics. The teacher is the real field worker, who knows what is most suitable and where. At present, the teacher is not consulted at all. The curriculum is laid down for him. He is to faithfully go through it, without any alteration or modification.

8. Some Other Requirements

(a) *Child centred Syllabus*: The curriculum should be child centred and not subject or topic-centred. Unless the requirement of the child are kept in view, the curriculum shall not be useful.

(b) *From Empirical to Rational*: The curriculum should be so organised that the students are able to acquire facts through experience, intuition and induction. They should also be gradually made to feel the need for and appreciate the usefulness of deduction system of education. This method is known as the method of proceeding from empirical to rational. In other words, it means that the students should be made to proceed from known to unknown or from particular to general.

(c) *From Concrete to Abstract:* The curriculum should provide for the teaching of the subject on the principle of proceeding from concrete to abstract.

4.6 GENERAL PATTERN OF SOCIAL STUDIES CURRICULUM

Some of the topics that may be included in the social studies curriculum for various classes are listed below. These are only suggestive and it is for the teachers and educators to make the final choice keeping in view the needs and capacities of the pupils, the needs of the community and other administrative considerations.

1. Family Environment

Individual in relation to family, contributions of individuals to the family, mutual help, respect and cooperation, rights and obligations of children and parents, family as a cradle of social and civic virtues.

2. Basic Human Needs and their Satisfaction

The way man satisfies his needs of food, clothing, shelter, transport, communication, power, education, religion, recreation etc.

3. Physical Environment

Soil, rain, sun, natural situation, weather, water resources, animal life, man's adjustment to physical environment.

4. Social Environment

Human relationships, village, town, school, games, fairs, festivals, farms, shops and factories. Inter-dependence of man and man. Man's adjustment to social order.

5. Cultural Environment

Personal hygiene, good manners, religious and social customs, stories of ancient heroes and heroines, Ancient Indian culture and civilization and its impact at present.

6. Economic Environment

Occupations of people, agriculture, industries, money transaction, production, distribution and exchange of things and goods. Raising standard of living, problem of unemployment and various possible solutions for these.

7. Political and Civic Environment

Citizenship, rights and duties. Civic sense and responsibility. Need for security and protection. Local Government, Village Panchayat, and Municipal Committee. Tehsil, District, State and National Administration, Institutions under the government and their utility.

8. Impact of Science and Technology of Man

Science in the service of man. Life-stories of famous scientists and inventors. Man's conquest of time, distance, water and air. Technology in agricultural and industrial development.

9. Current Problems that Confront Modern Man

Individual citizen in relation to world community. Need for world-peace and international understanding. The U.N.O. and the Panch-Shila. International trade and commerce. Interdependence of nation and nation.

10. Activities

Different types of sharing, experience-getting and knowledge-getting activities, including the preparation of charts, models, pictures and maps, group discussions, dramatisation, surveys, visits and excursions, and celebration of national and international days.

While selecting topics for syllabus to be introduced in different grades, the natural plan should be to start from the *immediate known to the distant unknown*. In other words, we should proceed from the direct experiences of children to the generalised concepts. For example, if in Junior and Primary classes we teach "Home duties and obligations of parents and children," in Senior or Middle classes we may explain "Family, as a social and civic institution." Similarly, if in Junior classes we teach "Soil, sun, rain and weather," in senior classes we may widen the horizon of pupils by teaching them how physical environment affects lives and occupations of people. From the "home and neighbourhood" we have to take the child to his state, his country and even beyond. This will gradually give him a sense of "community living", in larger and larger groups till he reaches the "world community." In this way there shall be a certain amount of duplication and repetition under different heads, but it is essential.

4.7. CURRICULUM OF SOCIAL STUDIES FOR VARIOUS STAGES OF EDUCATION

Normally speaking we have five stages of education. These are:

(i) Pre-primary

(ii) Primary

(iii) Junior High School (Middle)

(iv) Secondary/Senior Secondary

(v) University.

There is need to have a properly organised curriculum of various stages of education. Outline syllabus of various stages is as follows:

Syllabus or Curriculum at the Pre-primary and Primary Stage of Education

This is the stage where the children between the age 4 to 11 years come for education. This education runs upto V class. At this stage of education the main aim is to develop in the students the basic qualities of human life. The syllabus of social studies for this stage of education should be of an elementary nature. It should be based on certain elementary principles of formation of good habits and imparting knowledge of necessary requirements of life.

Prayer, healthy living, knowledge about school, festivals of social and cultural importance, gardening, knowledge about crops, postal facilities, life in the locality, important places of cultural and emotional value should form the subject-matter of social studies.

Curriculum Approach at the Primary Stages

The Curriculum for Ten Years (1976) has observed that the primary concern of the school at this stage should be to develop the necessary social skills, values and attitudes that would enable the child to contribute his mite, as he grows, towards the development of the society to which he belongs.

During the five years of primary school the child's mental horizon would be gradually widened from the home to the school and the local community to the world. In the process, the child would begin to appreciate the geographical elements of his environment. Various human activities, which help him to understand how the gifts of nature are processed to produce goods for serving the various needs of man, would also be studied. He would also get an idea of the social and cultural life in different parts of the country as well as of some different ways of living, in certain parts of the world. Stories and narratives about personages and events that have contributed to our national heritage and human heritage will also be studied. In addition to these, the child would get ample opportunities to develop socially desirable habits, attitudes and values besides becoming broadly acquainted with the functioning of political and social institutions.

To provide the pupils practical experiences actual real life situations be created in the schools. In the words of All India Council for Secondary Education, "The Class-room must function as a natural laboratory for social and democratic living. Students should spend time on the solution of real life problems, assume individual and group responsibilities for managing some aspects of school-life and work and cooperate in desirable community activities."

At this stage practical training in clean and orderly habit should be given through various activities, visits to fields, factories, mills and places where articles of food, cloth and shelter are produced should be organised in groups. At later stages trips to places of historical and social interest may be organised occasionally during the year. During these trips practical training be given in crossing roads safely and in walking on roads and streets in an orderly and safe manner. Practical training should be given in reading maps of the locality and the district and locating important places therein. If possible the activities such as collection of stamps, pictures, coins, newspaper cuttings, specimens of clothes, numerals etc., may be encouraged.

The syllabus in Social Studies at the primary stage should concentrate on the environment of child. The suggested syllabus for this stage is as follows:

1. Physical Aspects

(a) The sun, rain, weather, season, directions, soil and rivers, oceans, mountains, natural resources and their effect on man's life.

(b) The role of physical environment in making available to us the necessities of life.

(c) Physical features of the village or town (Class II), district (Class III), State (class IV) and India (Class V). The effect of the physical features on lives of the people.

(d) Lives of people in some region of the world.

2. Economical Aspect

(a) Man's economic activities, farming and agriculture, various occupations, handicrafts, industries and trade.

(b) Exchange of things, village and town markets; Important "**mandies**" of the state, Bank and their functions, cooperative societies.

(c) Means of communication and transport in the village, town and in the state, expansion of human relationship.

(d) Importance of animals in our economic life.

3. Historical and Cultural Aspect

(a) Personal hygiene, personal cleanliness of environment—home, school, neighbourhood, village or town.

(b) Good manners, religious and social customs, celebration of festivals.

(c) Stories of important personalities of India, from ancient times to modern age, in chronological order, their contribution to social and cultural life.

4. Social Aspect

(a) Man, a social animal; social life in families, schools, neighbourhood, village or town, at state level and at national level.

(b) Stories of food, shelter and clothing.

(c) Social institutions like families, schools, clubs, organisations.

(d) Influence of religion on social life.

5. Civic and Political Aspect

(a) Home, the cradle of civic and social virtue, rights and duties of parents and children.

(b) Our duties as citizens of free India towards our neighbours in the village, district, state, country and beyond.

(c) Political institutions like Panchayat, Municipal Committee. Zila Parishad, State Assembly and Union Government and their important functions for providing various amenities.

6. Current Problems

(a) Road safety, fight against disease, hunger, ignorance, dirt and idleness.

(b) Social welfare and community development programme.

(c) Five Year Plans in the context of the state.

(d) Study of current events through daily news papers, according to the standard of pupils.

Syllabus at the Junior High School Stage of Education (Middle School Stage)

Here the course is of three years. The aim of education is to bring about the development of the physical and mental faculties of the students. A tendency to acquire knowledge and make discoveries about things is developing in the students. An attempt is made to integrate the teaching of Social Studies with the teaching of other subjects. Attempt is also make to teach the practical aspect of the Social Studies. The principles of Social Studies can very well be applied in the school life. The students can also be shown the working of the theory in the world outside the school. In fact, the real aim of teaching Social Studies is to help the students to understand the elements of their social atmosphere, local life and their (political and cultural) aspect of the society. The syllabus of the Junior High Schools is as given below:

1. Physical Aspects

(a) Earth and its place in the solar system, rotation and revolution, change of season, external and internal agents of change and their effects on the lives of people, climatic effects.

(b) Broad features of life in major natural regions of the world.

(c) Geographical and commercial position of India, its physical features, climate, forest production and numerical resources. Flora and Fauna. Life and occupation of people in various parts of India. Effect of physical environment on the life and occupation of people. Means of communication and transport. The chief ocean, land and air routes of the world with special reference to India. Inland trade and trade of India with other countries. Distribution of articles of food, clothing and shelter on national and international level.

2. Economic Aspect

Satisfaction of human wants, India towards self-sufficiency in many respects, use of machines on agricultural farms and in factories. Economic development through Five Year Plans. Dependence on other countries. Economic interdependence of the nations of the world.

3. Historical and Cultural Aspect

(a) Primitive man and his struggle against nature to secure better life. Early movements and settlements of races. Aryan civilization.

(b) A brief outline of the main stages of the development of Indian culture through the ages. Impact and contribution of Greeks, Muslims, Christians, Modern culture and the impact of the West. Personalities of the country who shaped the past and the present India.

(c) Modern civilization, a world product.

4. Social Aspect

Group life and social relationship. Social life in different periods of Indian history. Present social conditions of the people of India. Uplift of socially backward classes.

5. Civic and Political Aspect

Organisation of community life. Understanding of mutual interdependence in home, school, business and society. Govt. of the home. Local Self-Government in village and town. Zila Parishad, the State and Union Governments and their organs. Law-making for security and justice. How our Government raises and spends money for our welfare? Education for citizenship. Responsibilities of a democratic citizen on national and international level.

6. Current Problems

(a) India's foreign policy and Panchshila.

(b) Five Year Plans on National basis.

(c) National integration.

(d) Multipurpose projects and schemes.

(e) Study of current problems through daily newspapers according to the standard of pupils.

7. Effects of modern science and technology on political, social and cultural life.

Syllabus at the Secondary Stage of Education

When the student reaches this stage of education he has already acquired some maturity. His mental powers such as imagination, reasoning, power of determination, etc. have developed by now. The students have also, by this time, learnt the art of shouldering the responsibilities. They now try to understand various social, political, religious and cultural problems. These things need that the syllabus at this stage of education should be scientific and properly organised. It should be competent to develop the students into ideal citizens of democratic republic.

Aims and Objectives of Teaching Social Studies at the Secondary Stage of Education

At this stage of education the teaching of Social Studies should aim at the following:

1. To develop the spirit of sacrifice, co-operation, love, etc. among the students so that they may try to lead the life of an ideal citizen.
2. The students should be acquainted with the democratic system of government of the State. This shall encourage them to take interest in the working of the government.
3. The student should be given an idea of the complex structure of the society and various social problems. They should be given an opportunity to observe various events and objects. Such a step will develop the spirit of patriotism in the students. This patriotism and nationalism shall be in co-existence with internationalism.
4. The students should be given a practical idea of the government, by practising it, on a miniature stage, in the school.
5. An attempt should be made to acquaint the students with the problems, of the country. Qualities of national con-

sciousness, emotional integration, co-operation, equality etc. should be developed in them.

Social Studies as an integrated subject be taught only in Classes IX and X and in classes XI and XII specialised study in history, geography, civics, economics, and sociology be taken up as separate subjects. For classes IX and X the syllabus for social studies should be as follows:

1. Physical Aspects

(a) Major natural regions of the world and their chief characteristics.

(b) Physical feataures, climatic conditions and natural resources of India. Main agricultural and industrial activities of the people of India. Influence of physical features on occupations of the people, internal and external trade and means of communication and transport in the country.

(c) Major sea, land and air routes of the world with special reference to India.

2. Economic Aspect

(a) Challenge of machinery to cottage industries; problem of nationalisation of production; different plans and projects of our country. The community development projects.

(b) Agricultural development for feeding India's increasing population.

(c) Industrial development for raising standard of living and progress of heavy industries.

(d) Economic inter-dependence of the nations of the world.

(e) Vinoba's philosophy and socialistic pattern of society.

3. Historical and Cultural Aspect

(a) Birth of life on the earth, the evolution of life and the coming of man. Man's conquest over nature, the hunting stage, the use of fire, the birth of language, the pastoral stage, the agricultural stage.

(b) Life in pre-historic and ancient times, River-Valley civilizations: the Greek, the Roman and the Aryan civilizations.

(c) Ancient Indian civilization. Impact and contribution of Islam to Indian Culture. The influence of the West on India.

(d) The growth of national consciousness in India, with important events leading upto the establishment of the Republic.

(e) Modern civilization, a world product.

4. Social Aspect

(a) Living as citizens of free India.

(b) Post-independent social problems and their solution. Gandhian way of life. India as a welfare state.

5. Civic and Political Aspect

Problems of present democracy in the world. The twoworld wars and the need for peace. The U.N.O. and its agencies. India's contribution to world peace. The Panch-Shila.

6. Current Problems

(a) National integration and internal peace.

(b) Beggar problem.

(c) Prohibition.

(d) International understanding.

(e) Study of current national and international problems through daily newspapers.

7. Effects of advances in Science and Technology on modern life.

Social Science Syllabus Prescribed by N.C.E.R.T. for Upper Primary or Middle Classes

History — Class VI — Ancient India

Unit I	(a) How and Why We study the Past. (b) Geographical and Ethnographical Features of India. (c) Pre-historic Culture of India.
Unit II	The Harrppa culture.
Unit III	New Cultural Patterns in India (1500 B.C. to 600 B.C.).

Unit IV	India from the Rise of Magadha to the Mauryan Empire.
Unit V	India during the Period 200 B.C. to 300 A.D.
Unit VI	India from 300 A.D. to 800 A.D.

Class VII — Medieval India

Unit I	India and the World
Unit II	India from 800 A.D. to 1200 A.D.
Unit III	India from Early 13th to early 16th Century.
Unit IV	Advent of the Mughals and Europeans.
Unit V	India under the Mughals.
Unit VI	Disintegration of the Mughal Empire.

Class VIII — Modern India

Unit I	India and the Modern World.
Unit II	The Rise, Growth and Impact of British Rule in India.
Unit III	Revolts against British Rule.
Unit IV	British Policies and Administration in India atter 1858.
Unit V	Changes in Economy and Society.
Unit VI	Rise of Indian Nationalism and Struggle for Freedom, upto Independence.

Geography — Class VI

Unit I	The Earth — Our Planet
Unit II	Africa — Lands and People.
Unit III	South America — Lands and People.
Unit IV	Australia — Land and People.
Unit V	Antarctica — Land, Climate, Natural Vegetation and Wild Life.
Unit VI	Practical Work — Map Reading.

Class VII

Unit I	Atmosphere and Hydrosphere.
Unit II	North America — Lands and Peoples.
Unit III	Europe — Lands and People.
Unit IV	The Soviet Union — Land and People.
Unit V	Practical Work — Studying the weather and night-sky.

Class VIII

Unit I	Lithosphere and Land forming.
Unit II	Asia — Lands and People.
Unit III	India — Physical Setting.
Unit IV	India — Natural Resources.
Unit V	India — Human Resources.
Unit VI	India — Economic Development.
Unit VII	Practical Work — Studying Local Maps.

Civics — Class VI

Unit I	Civic Life in the Community Development of the Community.
Unit II	Local Government Rural.
Unit III	Local Government Urban.
Unit IV	District Administration.
Unit V	Preservation of Property of the Community.
Unit VI	Project Work.

Class VII — Our Constitution

Unit I	Features of Our Constitution.
Unit II	Law Making Process.
Unit III	Executing Laws.

Unit IV	Interpreting Laws.
Unit V	Project Work.

Class VIII - Independent India — Achievements and Challenges

Unit I	Our National Goals.
Unit II	Strengthening the Democracy.
Unit III	Our Social Problems.
Unit IV	Our Economic Problems.
Unit V	National Integration.
Unit VI	Defence of the Country.
Unit VII	India and the World.
Unit VIII	World Problems (a) Arms Race, (b) Disparities between Developing and Developed Countries, (c) Environmental Pollution.
Unit IX	Project Work.

Social Science Syllabus Prescribed by N.C.E.R.T. New Delhi for Secondary Classes (IX and X)

History

Semester I

Unit I	Preliminary Stage.
Unit II	Bronze Age Civilizations.
Unit III	Early Iron Age Societies (1200 B.C. to 600 A.D.).
Unit IV	Early African and American Cultures and Civilizations.
Unit V	The Medieval World.

Semester II

Unit VI	Beginning of the Modern Age.
Unit VII	Capitalism and the Industrial Revolution.
Unit VIII	Revolutionary and Nationalist Movements.
Unit IX	Imperialism.

Semester III

Unit X	The First World War.
Unit XI	The Russian Revolution.
Unit XII	The World from 1919 to the Second World War.
Unit XIII	The World after the Second World War.
Unit XIV	The Cultural Heritage of India.
Unit XV	Indian Awakening.
Unit XVI	India's Struggle for Freedom, upto Independence.

Geography

Semester I

Unit I	Map Skills.
Unit II	Natural Environment.
Unit III	Natural Resources and their Utilization.

Semester II

Unit IV	Human Interaction with the Environment.

Semester III

Unit V	India, Physical features, Climate, Natural Vegetation and Wild Life.
Unit VI	Natural Resources.

Semester IV

Unit VII	Developing our Resources.
Unit VIII	Field study Project Work.

Civics

Semester I

Unit I	Man as a Citizen.
Unit II	Government at Local Level.
Unit III	Government at the State and National Levels.

Semester II

Unit IV India as a Nation.

Unit V Indian Democracy at Work.

Unit VI Challenges Facing our Country Today.

Unit VII India and World Peace.

Economics

Semester I

Unit I Understanding an Economy.

Unit II An overview of the Indian Economy.

Semester II

Unit III Infrastructure of the Indian Economy.

Unit IV Towards Economic Development.

Unit V State as an Agency for Economic Development.

Appraisal and Critical Observation

Although the syllabus in Social Sciences, prescribed by N.C.E.R.T. for Secondary Classes, is not free from certain flaws, it is, to a great extent, a very satisfactory attempt and is in accordance with the latest demands of Indian education. In this syllabus, the principle of integrated course has been accepted while recognising the existence of its constituent subjects, holds the needs and interests of students, along the logical demands of subject-matter. It includes a lot of practical work, in the shape of activities, field surveys, tours and trips, map-reading and map-making, project work, collection of cartoons, newspaper cuttings and pictures, preparation of time lines, graphs and charts and maintaining a record book, etc.

The following are some of the drawbacks of this syllabus:

The syllabus is dominated by History which occupies the most important place in the syllabus prescribed for various classes. In Middle Classes, the whole of History of India, from pre-historic times upto the present days, has been prescribed. In high classes world history from the "Evolution of Life on Earth" upto the World after the Second World War, together with the British Occupation of India, Indian Awakening and India's Struggle for Freedom, has been prescribed. It also includes the study of all the ancient world civilizations, early African and American civilizations as also the civilizations of medieval Europe, Arabia and East Asia. It also includes the world revolutionary movements, like the American Revolution, the French Revolution and the Russian Revolution etc., for high classes.

Traditionalism dominates the syllabus. Large portions of history, geography, civics and economics have been included in the syllabus under separate unit-heads. It is simply a combination of various subjects and not psychological integration of material, as recommended by the N.C.E.R.T. itself. It says, "The various components, drawn from different social sciences, should not, however, be seen as isolated components, but as being inter-related." This combination of different subjects has made the syllabus lengthy and monotonous. It is not possible to finish the whole of the syllabus, meant for each class, in one academic year, when generally five periods a week are allotted to the teaching of social sciences, in the time table.

REVISION QUESTIONS

1. Give a general pattern of contents to be included in Social Studies curriculum for various classes.
2. Give a critical observation of NCERT syllabus, prescribed for secondary classes.
3. Discuss the need, importance and main purposes of a Social Studies Curriculum.
4. Do we actually require a curriculum for instruction in Social Studies? If so, what purpose is it expected to serve?
5. What place would you give to social studies in Junior and Senior High School syllabus? Draw up briefly a syllabus for the same.
6. What do you understand by the term 'curriculum'? What is the need for planning the curriculum?

5

Methods of Teaching Social Studies

5.1 INTRODUCTION

A *teaching method* is nothing but a way of imparting knowledge to the students.

For teacher of every subject method is important. Method is nothing but a *scientific way of presenting the subject, keeping in mind the psychological and physical requirements of the children.* There may be more than one method of teaching, as there are more than one road for going to a destination. We have to select a method out of various methods of teaching. While selecting a method we have to keep in mind the psychology of the students, their interests, mental aptitudes and other mental faculties. In Social Studies we make an effort to acquaint the child with the basic elements of ideal citizenship. In order to help the students to attain this goal, various methods are employed. It has rightly been said by Bining and Bining:

> "Methodology should be conceived as a dynamic function of education and not as a static aspect of the process of teaching."

To quote the Secondary Education Commission, "Any method, good or bad links up the teacher and his pupils into an organic relationship with constant mutual interaction. It reacts not only on the mind of the students but on their entire personality; their standard of work and judgement, their intellectual and emotional development, their attitudes and values. Good methods which are psychologically and socially sound may raise the whole quality of life; bad methods debase it. So, in the choice and assessment of methods, teachers must always take into consideration their end products, namely the attitudes and values inculcated in them consciously and unconsciously."

Further emphasising the need for right methods, the Secondary Education Commission states, "Every teacher and educationist experiences or knows that even the best curriculum and the most perfect syllabus remain dead unless quickened into life by the right method of teaching and the right kind of teacher. Sometimes even an unsatisfactory and unimaginative syllabus can be made interesting and significant by the gifted teacher who does not focus his mind or the subject-matter to be taught or the information to the imparted but on his students — their interests and aptitudes, their reaction and response. He judges the success of his lesson not the amount of matter covered but by the understanding, the appreciation and the efficiency achieved by the students."

In order to make children learn effectively the teacher has to adopt the right method of teaching.

5.2 VARIOUS METHODS OF TEACHING SOCIAL STUDIES

With the development of the subject-matter and knowledge of Social Studies, various methods have evolved and are used for teaching of social studies. Some of the important methods of teaching of Social Studies are:

1. Text-book Method
2. Lecture Method
3. Observation Method
4. Project Method
5. Unit Method
6. Laboratory Method
7. Activity Method
8. Problem solving Method
9. Source Method.
10. Recitation or Socialised Recitation Method
11. Survey Method
12. Dramatic Method
13. Comparative Method
14. Narration Method or Method of Narration

Important Characteristics of a Good Teaching Method

1. They should aim at inculcating 'love of work'.
2. They should aim to develop the desire for doing work with the highest measure of efficiency of which one is capable. The motto of every school and its pupils should be "everything that is worth doing at all is worth doing well." Whether it be making a speech, writing a composition, drawing a map, cleaning the classroom, making a book rack or forming a queue.
3. They should provide various opportunities of free participation in accepted projects and activities wherein discipline and co-operation are constantly in demand.
4. They should aim at developing the capacity for 'clear-thinking' which distinguishes every truly educated person, "whether a student is asked to make a speech in a debating society or to write an essay or to answer a question in history, geography, or science or to experiment, the accent should always be on clear thinking and on lucid expression which is a mirror of clear thought."
5. The methods of teaching should expand the range of students interest. "We would urge all schools to provide in the time-table, at least one free period every day in which student may puruse their favourite hobbies and creative activities individually or in groups, preferably under the guidance of some interest teacher," recommended the Secondary Education Commission.
6. They should aim at providing opportunities to pupils to apply practically the knowledge that has been acquired by them. They should aim at transforming present bookish schools into work "schools" or "activity schools."
7. They should aim at the quickening of interest and training in efficient techniques of learning and study.
8. They should train the students in the art of study. They should train the students in the use of reference material such as the list of contents and index in books, the dictionary, the atlas, and reference books like the encyclopaedia.

9. They should be adapted to suit different levels of intelligence.
10. They should be such as they balance the claim of individual work with co-operative or group effort. The training of emotions, attitudes and social capacities take place best in the context of projects and units of work undertaken co-operatively. The Secondary Education Commission has recommended that the teachers should be so trained that they are able to visualise and organise at least a part of the curriculum in the form of projects and activity-units which groups of students may take up and carry to completion.

Since methods are closely related to aims and objectives of teaching a particular subject, so before determining the procedure let us have a fresh look at the major specific aims of teaching Social Studies. These are:

(i) the acquisition of knowledge and concepts; and
(ii) the development of attitudes and skills.

Corresponding to these major aims of teaching, there are two ways of learning social studies:

(i) learning through the subject of matter; and
(ii) learning through organised situation and experiences.

For the former, the Text-book Method, the Lecture Method and the Discussion Method are considered to be most suitable. For the latter, the Project Method, the Problem Method, the Unit Method, the Source Method and the Socialized Recitation Method are thought to be most effective and beneficial.

We now take up a few of these methods:

1. Text-book Method

This is the method in which social studies is taught through text-books. Certain text-books are prescribed for the students. The teacher teaches social studies on the basis of those text books. It is more or less a direct method of teaching social studies. This method is being used in India for a long time. It cannot be called independent method. The teacher and taught both are bound down by the limitations of the text-book. According to E.B. Wesley it is an old method of teaching and the Text-book method may be defined as that teaching procedure in which is understanding of the main body of information in the text-book is the immediate objective. It means that this is the procedure which "revolves around the text-book just as another procedure might revolve around the problem or the project"[1]. However, within the limits of the text-book method, we may find good as well as bad teaching. Since the text-book is very widely used, it is highly desirable on the part of the teacher to utilize it to the best advantage of his pupils.

Text-book is a very useful means of getting concise and uptodate information. An oral lesson on the other hand, may become lengthy, complicated and unintelligible. In a text-book, the subject-matter is logically and systematically arranged for students. As such, it gives the minimum essentials and enables them to work out problems and projects and also to pursue further discussion.

While adopting this method the teacher of social studies should make a judicious use of the text-book. He should consider text-book only as an effective aid. He should never depend on one text-book completely. He must consult other text-books, source books, reference books etc. to supplement the subject-matter given in anyone particular text-book. He should also tell his students how to make best use of the text book. For this he should give a demons-tration alongwith his comments and ask his students to follow in that manner.

Merits of Text-book Method

(i) It brings about efficiency and provides knowledge to the students. The text-books are written with the students in view and so they are useful for them. They develop in the students the habit of study as well as self-study.

(ii) They develop in the students the habit of doing work in a systematic and scientific manner. Books are written in a scientific and systematised manner and so it is possible for the students to have an idea of systematic work.

(iii) Since the students have to memorise the facts that are given in the books, their memory improves. Here Thorndike's law of learning operates.

1. Edgar Bruce Wesley, *Teaching Social Studies in High Schools,* p. 445.

(iv) Text-books give a reasonably correct account of the subject field or area in an organised manner.

(v) Text-books also suggest application of the subject-matter, through assignments, drills, questions, projects and other activities.

(vi) Text-book indicates what the teacher is required to teach and what the pupils are supposed to learn. It furnishes a definite basis of specific assignments, problems and projects.

(vii) A text-book can expand and delimit its scope, size and content according to the changing needs of education.

(viii) It is possible to adopt almost all other methods with the text-books as the basis of study.

(ix) A text-book presents history and current affairs in such a way as to help pupils to develop an appreciation of different points of view.

Limitations of Text-book Method

(i) This method does not employ or use the maxims and principles of education.

(ii) This method narrows the outlook of students and they become inactive and lethargic. They do not participate actively in the acquisition of knowledge.

(iii) In the method the scope of revision is very limited and the knowledge acquired by the student is not permanent.

(iv) A text-book because of its definite and convenient subject matter may dominate the entire procedure of teaching.

Conclusion

After considering the merits and limitations it may be concluded that too much reliance and emphasis upon the text-book should not be placed because text-book method is not a complete method in itself. Teacher should use this method in combination with other methods of teaching. Teacher should give assignments which should be challenging so as to motivate the pupils for self-activity in learning and self-study.

2. Lecture Method

Lecture method is the most commonly practised in teaching Social Studies. This method is most commonly followed in schools for teaching social studies to higher classes. It is also known as 'Telling of Story method' or "Conversational method."

In this method only the teacher talks and the students are the passive listeners. Since students do not actively participate in this method of teaching so this method is a teacher controlled and information centred. In this method teacher works as a sole resource in classroom instructions. Due to lack of participation students get bored and sometimes may go to sleep. In this method student is provided with readymade knowledge by the teacher and due to this spoon feeding the student loses interests and his power of reasoning and observation get no stimulus.

In this method teacher goes ahead with the subject-matter at his own speed. The teacher may make use of black-boards at times, and may also dictate notes. This teacher oriented method in its extreme form does not expect any questions or response from the students.

Advantages of Lecture Method

It has the following advantages:

(i) It is quite economical method. It is possible to handle a large number of students at a time and no laboratory equipment, aids, materials are required.

(ii) Using this method the knowledge can be imparted to the students quickly and the prescribed syllabus can be covered in short time.

(iii) It is quite attractive and easy to follow. Using this method teacher feels secure and satisfied.

(iv) It simplifies the task of the teacher as he dominates the lesson for 70-85% of lesson time and students just listen to him.

(v) Using this method it is quite easy to impart factual information and historical anecdotes.

(vi) By following this method teacher can develop his own style of teaching and exposition.

(vii) In this method teacher can easily maintain the logical sequence of the subject by planning his lectures in advance. It minimises the chances of any gaps or overlappings.

(viii) Some good lectures delivered by the teacher motivate, instigate, inspire a student for some creative thinking.

(ix) Since lecture method demands a lot of preparation on the part of the teacher, its advantages are transferred to the class as a whole. Teacher, own preparation, his enthusiasm and his interest do stimulate good students who may therefore like to pursue projects, problems and other such activities in order to gain more and more knowledge.

This method may, however be used with advantage only on suitable occassions for:

(a) *Stimulating students*

(b) *Classifying concepts*

(c) *Supplementing the knowledge of pupils*

(d) *Summing up the findings of the pupils*

(e) *Preparing the students to undertake an assignment, a project or an activity.*

Disadvantages of Lecture Method

The disadvantages of lecture method can be as under:

(i) In this method the student's participation is negligible and students become passive recipients of information.

(ii) In this method we are never sure if the students are concentrating and understanding the subject-matter being taught to them by the teacher.

(iii) In this method knowledge is imparted so rapidly that weak students develop a hatred for learning.

(iv) It does not allow all the faculties of the student to develop.

(v) In this method there is no place of 'learning by doing'.

(vi) It does not take into account the previous knowledge of the student.

(vii) It does not provide for corrective feedback and remedial help to slow learners.

(viii) It does not cater to the individual needs and differences of students.

(ix) It does not keep to inculcate scientific attitudes and training in scientific method among the pupils.

(x) It is an undemocratic and authoritarian method in which students depend only on the authority of the teacher. They cannot challenge or question the verdict of the teacher. This checks the development of power of critical thinking and proper reasoning in the student.

Conclusion

After considering various merits and demerits of method it may be concluded that this method may be suitable for teaching in higher classes (XI, XII) where we aim to cover the prescribed syllabus quickly. In these classes this method can be used successfully for imparting factual knowledge, introducing some new and difficult topics, make generalisation from the facts already known to the students, revision of lessons already learnt etc.

Teaching by this method the students of classes XI and XII will also help those students who intend to join college so that they can prepare themselves for college where lecture method of teaching is a dominant method of imparting instructions.

This method of teaching can be made more beneficial if the teacher encourages his students to take notes during the lesson. After the lesson teacher can give to his students sometime for asking questions and answer their questions without any hesitation. While delivering his lesson the teacher may see that the lesson is delivered in good tone, loudly and clearly. He should use only simple and understandable words for delivering his lesson. If teacher can introduce some humour in his lesson it would keep students interested in his lesson.

The teacher of social studies may utilize this method profitably for:

(i) giving background of a topic,

(ii) giving an over-view of a large unit,

(iii) create interest in the pupils, and

(iv) explaining and correcting some faulty ideas or introducing an intelligent assignment.

3. Observation Method

Students travel from one place to another during tours and while going from one place to another they get an opportunity to observe and see things for themselves. A real impression of an object or a place can best be gained through personal observation. Direct experience is an essential step to right understanding. If the students are given an opportunity to acquire knowledge of social studies by observing things themselves the knowledge shall be stable and shall have a practical value. The knowledge acquired through this method is clear, complete and prefect.

It is most desirable that observational work of the pupils be carefully directed and guided by the teacher. The students in lower classes may be asked to observe various things in their environment, near their homes, village and such other localities. They may be told to collect the relevant data. This data will help them understand similar conditions in their own provinces extending to other countries of the world. The observation method has a very wide range and can be very conveniently employed. The teacher does not play any part in this method. He remains a guide and a philosopher. No doubt he encourages the students to acquire knowledge.

This method may be used at any stage of education, best it is quite useful at primary and secondary stages of education.

Some of the important requirements of this method are as under:

(i) The teacher himself should have properly observed and seen things which he expects his students to see and observe. It is important because in the absence of a thorough knowledge of those things he will not be able to impart as scientific knowledge to his students.

(ii) Necessary data must be collected during observation.

Merits of the Observation Method

It has the following qualities in it:

(i) Here the students acquire knowledge independently. They remain active in the acquisition of knowledge and so the knowledge that is acquired, is stable and stands is good stead in future life.

(ii) This leads to the development of mental faculties of observation, reasoning, thinking etc.

(iii) It brings about a close co-operation in the school and the society.

(iv) The knowledge that is acquired by this method is acquired directly by the child.

Difficulties of the Method

(i) While on trips/tours the teacher sometimes has to face the problem of discipline.

(ii) The tours/trips cannot be planned to observe things that are situated far away.

(iii) Sometimes guardians are reluctant to permit their wards to go out for observation.

Precautions

Teacher, if he wants to use this method, should keep the following thing in his mind:

(i) Here the teacher asks his students to observe a thing, he should himself observe it. This will help the teacher to guide his students properly.

(ii) The teacher should act as an alert guide. No doubt, students should be given freedom to observe things but while giving them freedom, he should keep an eye on them so that they may not go astray.

(iii) Observation should not be passive. The teacher should continue to ask questions to the students so that they may go on understanding the things that they have observed.

(iv) The task of the teacher does not finish with the observation. He should test whether the students have really acquired knowledge or not.

(v) The teacher should try to ask the students to write down what they have observed. This will give a stable base to the knowledge.

4. Discussion and Debate Method

This method is said to be very useful to the study of social studies. In this method the students are given certain problems and they are asked to discuss and debate them. They are themselves asked to prepare the outline of the discussions. Students prepare the discussions at home and they study the problems thoroughly well. This discussion may be on formal as well as informed lines. In this method the students get opportunity to express their ideas and feelings independently.

Essential Parts or Constituents of a Discussion

The essential parts of a discussion are (i) A leader, (ii) A group (iii) A problem, and (iv) A content.

(i) The Leader

In this method the teacher acts as a leader. To organise any discussion, teacher shall have to do a lot of study, preparation, selection and planning. However, teacher while acting as a leader, must not dominate the entire discussion. Teacher should act more as a guide when pupil face certain difficulties during discussion.

(ii) The Group

The students of the class will form the group. The teacher should see that each one from the group participates in discussion.

(iii) *The Problem*

The topic of discussion which is called the problem should be such that students feel it their own. The problem should be made as precise and exact as is possible. The problem be selected by the teacher with the active co-operation of the students. The problem that is selected should be real and functional and within capacity and comprehension of the pupils.

(iv) The Content

The content is the body of knowledge, the needed material of study. It should also include maps, charts, pictures, diagrams and other audio-visual aids. We cannot discuss facts but proposition, which are "statements about values" can be discussed and their truth established. It is about these statements that opinions may differ which may lead to a discussion.

Evaluation

After the discussion in over each participant should evaluate whether discussion about that particular problem or topic has added to his knowledge and information, changed his ideas, attitudes and prejudice and increased the range of his interest. A successful discussion must bring in the necessary change and make the participant a more active citizen than before.

Real Nature of a Discussion

It should be remembered that class-room discussion is not an occasion for practising the art of public speaking or skill in debating. "The debater always tries to win an argument. He knows no compromise. Discussion, on the other hand, is a sharing and weighing of all sides, which may be as many as there are conflicting interests or values." The participants in a discussion are inter-related in "a process of competitive co-operation". Agreement is the declared purpose of a discussion. It is always organised and undertaken in a disciplined atmosphere. Discussion is an important means of exchanging ideas with others and "often results in pooling opinions and joint action." A good discussion, in fact, is well-planned and well-mannered conversation. As such, every participant in a discussion, must be courteous, clear, good-natured, tolerant and sincere.

Merits of Discussion and Debate Method

(i) In this method, the students are faced with the problems, as they shall have to face in life.

(ii) By this method the defects of the classroom teaching may be removed and the students may be made active partners in the process of the education.

(iii) In this method the students themselves acquire knowledge and so the knowledge is stable and permanent.

(iv) This gives a chance to the students to solve their personal and individual problems. They learn a practical way of life.

(v) It leads to the development of the mental faculties of thinking, reasoning, determination, etc.

(vi) In discussion, the students have to present their ideas in a systematic manner. In doing so, they learn the art of systematising and organising their ideals properly. This is a great boon for future life.

(vii) This method inculcates tolerence. Different people may believe in the same thing differently for different reasons. Participants in a discussion must have the patience to listen to divergent opinion, and tolerate arguments contrary to their own.

Conclusion

One should always remember that this is not the **only** method of teaching social studies though it is one of the methods. This method is successful with grown up students under the guidance of a capable and hard working teacher.

5. Project Method

This method was given by Dewey — the American philosopher, psychologist and practical teacher. The project method is a direct outcome of his philosophy. According to Dr. Kilpatrick, "A project is a unit of whole-hearted purposeful activity carried on preferably, in its natural setting." According to Stevenson "A project is a problematic act carried to its completion in its natural setting." According to Ballard, "A project is a bit of real life that has been incorporated into the school."

In Burton's words, "The problem is a project which results in doing. The motor element is not what makes the activity a project, but the problem solving of a particular nature, accompanying the activity."

According to C.V. Good, "A project is a significant unit of activity, having educational value and aimed at one or more definite goals of understanding. It involves investigation and solution of problem and frequently the use and manipulation of physical materials. It is planned and carried to completion by the pupils and the teacher in a natural life-like manner."

From the above definitions it becomes clear that project method lays great stress on the actual action or activity on the part of the pupils. In this method, the curriculum, content and techniques of teaching are considered from the child's point of view. Thus "**Learning by Living**" is a better description of the project method than "learning by doing."

The project method is not totally new. Project equivalents are advocated for the adolescent period by Rousseau in Emile (BK-III). A project plan is modified form of an old method called "concentration-of-studies." The main features of "concentration-of-studies plan" is that some subject is taken the core or centre and all other school subjects as they arise are studied in connection with it.

Project method is based on the following principles:

(i) Learning by doing.

(ii) Learning by living.

(iii) Children learn better through association, co-operation and activity.

In this method, a project is taken, which is then completed in a natural and social setting. As the project is carried to completion, the students learn so many things.

Basic Principles of Project Method

This method is based on the following principles:

(i) *Principle of Purpose:* In this method the pupil is clear of the purpose of doing things in the school and so he feels more interested in the work.

(ii) *The principle of activity:* In this method pupils are provided with ample opportunities to think and plan things independently and then carry out the project in cooperation with others.

(iii) *The principle of experience:* This method gives a lot of experience to the child to work in groups. He learns to cooperate with others and to share his interests and purposes. It provides him the experiences in cooperation, character building, practical democracy and citizenship.

(iv) *The Principle of Freedom:* To act and to participate in any activity should not be forced, such a desire should be spotaneous and it should grow out of students own needs and purposes. The pupils should be left to themselves and be allowed to choose the activity according to their powers and capacities.

(v) *The Principle of Reality:* The effort be made to create real life situations in the school.

(vi) *The Principle of Utility:* Any knowledge gained through activity should be useful and practical.

Procedure

Project method generally involves the following steps:

(i) *Providing a situation:* The teacher provides a situation wherein the students feel like working on certain projects.

(ii) *Choosing:* Then the pupils are helped to choose a project linked to their need.

(iii) *Planning:* Pupils then discuss how that project is to be executed? Steps of the procedure are planned and noted down.

(iv) *Executing:* The project is then executed as planned. Every body contributes his share of work.

(v) *Evaluating:* The project is then evaluated and the possible knowledge is reviewed.

(vi) *Recording:* The knowledge gained is then recorded for future reference.

What is an Educational Project?

Various definitions of project have already been considered. A modified definition of project is given by Tomas and Long. They define it as "a voluntary undertaking which involves constructive effort or thought and eventuates into objective results."

Considering various definitions of project we may consider it as a kind of life experience which is an outcome of a craving or desire of the pupils. This is a method of spontaneous and incidental teaching. "Learning by living" may be a better meaning of project method, because life is full of projects and individuals carry out these projects in their every day life.

The projects may broadly be classified as:

(i) Individual projects, and

(ii) Social projects.

Individual projects are to be carried out by individuals whereas social projects are carried out by a group of individuals.

Steps in a Project

For completing a project we have five stages in actual practice. These are:

(i) Providing a situation

(ii) Choosing and proposing.

(iii) Planning of the project.

(iv) Executing the project.

(v) Judging the project.

Recording the project is also essential.

(i) Providing a Situation

A project should arise out of a need felt by pupils and it should never be forced on them. It should be purposeful and significant. It should look important and must be interesting. For this the teacher should always be on the look out to find situation that arise and discuss them with students to discover their interests. Situations may be provided by different methods. Some such methods may include talking to students on the topics of common interest e.g., how did they spend their holidays, what did they see in Delhi etc.

(ii) Choosing and Proposing

From various definitions of an educational project we get the same underlying ideas (a) school tasks are to be as real and as purposeful as the task of wider life beyond the school walls. (b) they are of such a nature that the pupils is genuinely eager to carry them out in order to achieve a desirable and clearly realised aim.

According to Kilpatrick, "the part of the pupils and the part of the teacher, in most of the school work, depends largely on who does the proposing." The teacher should refrain from proposing any project otherwise the whole purpose of the method would be defeated. Teacher should only tempt the students for a particular project by providing a situation but the proposal for the project should finally come from students. The teacher must exercise guidance in selection of the project and if the students make an unwise choice, the teacher should tactfully guide them for a better project. The essentials of a good project are:

(i) It should have evident worth for the individual or the group that undertakes them.

(ii) The project must have a bearing on a great number of subjects and the knowledge acquired through it may be applicable in a variety of ways.

(iii) The project should be timely.

(iv) The project should be challenging.

(v) The project should be feasible.

It is for the teacher to see that the purpose of the project is clearly defined and understood.

(iii) Planning

The students be encouraged by the teacher to plan out the details of the project. In the process of planning teacher has to act only as a guide and he should give suggestions at times but actual planning be left to the students.

(iv) Execution

Once the project has been chosen and details of the project have been planned, the teacher should help the students in executing the project according to the plan. Since execution of a project is the longest step in project method so it needs a lot of patience on the part of the students and the teacher. During this step the teacher should carefully supervise the pupils in manipulative skills to prevent waste of materials and to guard accidents. The teacher should assign work to different students in accordance with their tastes, interests, aptitudes and capabilities. Teacher should see that every member of the group gets a chance to do something. Teacher should constantly check up the relation between the chalked out plans and the developing project and as far as possible 'at the spot' changes and modification be avoided. However, if such changes become unavoidable these should be noted and reasons explained for future guidance.

(v) Evaluation

The evaluation of the project be done both by the pupils and the teacher. The pupils estimate the qualities of what they have done before the teacher gives his evaluation. The evaluation of the project has to be done in the light of plans, difficulties in the execution and achieved results. Let the students have self-criticism and look through their own failings and findings. The step is very useful because as a result of the project, the pupils can know the values of the information, interest, skills and attitudes that have been modified by the project.

(vi) Record

A complete record of the project be kept by the students. The record should include everything about the project. It should include the proposal, plan and its discussion, duties allotted to different students and how far were they carried out by them. It should also include the details of places visited and surveyed, maps, etc., drawn guidance for future and all other possible details.

Role of Teacher

(i) In project method of teaching the role of a teacher is that of a guide, friend and philosopher.

(ii) He helps the students in solving their problems just like an elder brother.

(iii) He encourages his students to work collectively, amicably in the group.

(iv) He also helps his students to avoid mistakes.

(v) He makes it a point that each member of the group contributes some thing to the completion of the project and in this process helps the shy and weaker students to work along with their classmates.

(vi) If the students face failure during execution of some steps of the project the teacher should not execute any portion of the project but should only explain to his students the reasons of their failure and should suggest them some better methods or techniques that may be used by them next time for the success of the project.

(vii) During the execution step teacher also learn something.

(viii) Teacher should always remain alert and active during execution, step and see that the project goes to completion successfully.

(ix) During execution of the project teacher should maintain a democratic atmosphere.

(x) Teacher must be well-read and well-informed so that he can help the students to the successful completion of the project.

Merits of the Project Method

(i) It is a method of teaching based on psychological laws of learning. The education is related to child's life and he acquires it through meaningful activity.

(ii) It imbibes the spirit of co-operation as it is a co-operative venture. Teacher and students join in the project.

(iii) It stimulates interest in natural as also man-made situations. Moreover the interest is spontaneous and not under any compulsions.

(iv) The method provides opportunities for pupils of different tastes and aptitudes with in the framework of the same scheme.

(v) It upholds the dignity of labour.

(vi) It introduces democracy in education.

(vii) It brings about a close correlation between a particular activity and various subjects.

(viii) It is a problem solving method and places very less emphasis on cramming or memorising.

(ix) It helps to inculcate social discipline through joint activities of the teacher and the taught.

(x) A project can be used to arouse interest in a particular topic as it blends school life with outside world. It provides situations in which the students come in direct contact with their environment.

(xi) It develops self-confidence and self-discipline.

(xii) A project tends to illustrate the real nature of the subject.

(xiii) A project affords opportunity to develop keenness and accuracy of observation and produces a spirit of enquiry.

(xiv) It puts a challenge to the student and thus stimulates constructive and creative thinking.

(xv) It provides the students an opportunity for mutual exchange of ideas.

(xvi) This method helps the children to organise their knowledge.

Drawbacks of the Project Method

(i) Projects require a lot of time.

(ii) Though the method provides the student superficial knowledge of so many things it provides insufficient knowledge of some fundamental principles.

(iii) In the project planning and execution of the project the teacher is required to put in much more work in comparison to other methods of teaching.

(iv) The teacher has been assumed as master of all subjects which is practically not possible.

(v) Good text books on these lines have not yet been produced.

(vi) It is an expensive method, it involves tours, excursions, purchase of apparatus and equipment etc.

(vii) The method of organising instructions is unsystematised and thus the regular time table of work will be upset.

(viii) The method may fit those who cannot listen but it is very questionable if it has the same value for those who can listen.

(ix) The method leaves a gap in pupils, knowledge.

(x) It underestimates man's power of imagination which enables him to savour the full experience of another without the necessity of undergoing the experience himself.

(xi) Sometimes project may be too ambitious and beyond pupil's capacity to accomplish.

(xii) Larger project in hands of an unexperienced teacher lead to boredom.

(xiii) The education given by projects is likely to emphasise relationships in breadth than the depth.

Conclusion

The project method provides a practical approach to learning of both theoretical and practical problems. It is difficult of follow this method of a teaching, it would be better at least not to ignore the spirit of this method.

This method has been found to be more suitable for primary and middle classes and is of restricted use for high and higher secondary classes. This method may be tried alongwith formal classroom teaching without disturbing the school time-table. With this in view some projects may be undertaken by the students to be completed on certain fixed days of a week. Alternately first half of the day may be devoted to classroom teaching and the project work be carried out in the remaining half day. To help solve the problem of fund's shortage such project be chosen which are self-supporting. As it is not suitable for drill and continuous and systematic teaching. It is not very desirable to use it freely.

Examples of Projects in Social Studies

There are a large number of projects that can be used in teaching of social studies, e.g. field trips, school elections, making card board, clay or wood models of different objects, writing plays based upon a period of history, preparing scripts for radio programmes, writing a song or a poem inspired by a historical event, dramatising events, making displays for bulletin board, preparing pageants, arranging community surveys and starting a collection of stamps, pictures, specimens and other such things for the scrap-books and for the school museum.

6. Unit Method

This method is of foreign origin and is quite popular in the United States of America. Gestalt's psychological theories have played a vital role in the development of this method. In this method it is proposed to present the subject-matter for teaching as a whole. This method is based on the assumption that body is a co-ordinated unit of physical and biological units. In the words of Henry C. Morrison: "Unit is a comprehensive and significant aspect of the environment of an organised science and an art. This is intended to make the teaching easy and convenient. For the convenience of teaching, a subject-matter is divided into certain units."

Michaelies defines unit in Social Studies as "a carefully developed series of experiences, related to a particular topic and designed to contribute to the achievement of purposes of Social Studies."

Hanna, Hageman and Potter state that, "a unit is a purposeful learning experience, focussed upon some socially significant understanding which will modify the behaviour of the learner and enable him to adjust to a life situation more effectively."

According to C.V. Good, "Unit is a major sub-division of a course of study, a text-book or a subject field, particularly a sub-division in Social Studies, practical arts or sciences. It is an organization of various activities, experiences and types of learning around a central theme, problem or purpose, developed cooperatively by a group of pupils under teacher leadership. It involves planning, execution of plan and evaluation of results."

In Social Studies the vast subject-matter has to be organised in large divisions. Each such division is called a unit. A unit is thus, "the organisation of material in related groups, each large enough to be significant but small enough to be seen as a whole by the pupils."

The unit may be a **subject-matter unit** or an **experience unit**. **Unit** is an instructional device to give knowledge or experience or both. It is "an organised body of information and experiences designated to effect significant outcomes for the learner."

Some of the units in Social Studies course for secondary classes may be:

(i) Influence of the west on Indian life and civilisation.

(ii) Feeding India's increasing millions.

(iii) How British traders became rulers of India?

(iv) How our community meets its economic needs?

(v) Contribution of Islam to Indian civilization and culture.

Formation of Unit

Units are formed so as to facilitate learning. Their function is to challenge and guide the student through a learning experience. Like most learning devices, the unit is a growth, an evolution, rather than a creation. The following points should be kept in mind while forming units:

1. Units for lower classes should be shorter than those meant for higher classes.
2. Children's needs, interests, capacities and capabilities should always be kept in mind while selecting units for them. Thus units should, rather centre round the children's expanding interests.
3. A unit must have relationship to the whole course.
4. A unit must be comprehensive enough on which sufficient material may be available for its complete understanding.
5. A good unit should provide for the intellectual, social and emotional development of children, through the integration and correlation of their learning activities.
6. A good unit should be evolutionary and functional, moving towards some definite goal.
7. Each unit should be further split up into sub-units for the sake of clarity. For example, the unit "How British Traders became Rulers of India" may be divided into the following sub-units:
   (i) Early European settlements and emergence of the British as the leading power.
   (ii) Decline of the Mughal Empire.
   (iii) Rise and Fall of the Marathas.
   (iv) Rise and Fall of Hyder Ali and Tippu.
   (v) Rise and Fall of Sikhs.

Steps of Unit

Morrison has laid down the following five steps of a unit:

1. *Exploration:* Under this procedure the students are prepared for a new unit. An attempt is made to explore their past knowledge.

2. *Presentation:* At this stage, the teacher through lecture and narration tries to present an outline of the unit to be presented before the students.
3. *Assimilation:* Under this heading, the students try to own and acquire the information that is provided to them.
4. *Recording:* At this stage the students try to organise the information that they have assimilated.
5. *Recitation:* At this stage, the students try to express in form of a lecture or action that they have acquired.

These stages cannot be determined from before hand. They grow out of the contact between the students and the teacher.

Merits of the Unit Method

This method has the following merits:

1. This creates in the students for the subject.
2. It is based on the idea of giving whole knowledge to the students and tries to remove the shyness of the students.
3. The students are taught to draw up plans of action. This drawing up of plans is helpful for their future life.
4. It is based on individual differences and develops in the students the habit of self-study.
5. The students are taught the lesson of carrying out their duties sincerely and shouldering the responsibilities properly.
6. It develops, in the students, the qualities of sympathy, love, tolerance, leadership, discipline, etc.

Limitations of Unit Method

In spite of the merits present in this method critics have pointed out certain defects as well. They are being enumerated below:

1. It is not useful for all subjects.
2. It does not train the students in the art of appreciation and does not develop only the aesthetic quality.
3. It is a very expensive method and consumes a lot of time.

4. Since the method lays stress on imparting knowledge of the whole to the students, so either the students acquire a whole knowledge or do not acquire any knowledge at all.

7. Dalton Plan or Laboratory Method

Origin and Significance of Daltan Plan: This method was given by Miss Helen Parkurst but it is not named after her. It is named after the town where it was adopted for the first time for teaching in a high school. It is also called Laboratory Plan because writing about the importance of word, 'Laboratory', Miss H. Parkurst says, "I cling to it in the hope that it may gradually shift the educational point of view away from the atmosphere of prejudice which the word 'School' calls up in our mind. Let us think school rather as a sociological laboratory where the pupils themselves are the experiments, not the victim of an intricate and crystallised system in the evolution of which they have neither part nor lot. Let us think of it as a place where community conditions prevail as they prevail in life itself."

Principles Underlying Dalton Plan

This method of teaching is based on the following principles:

(i) The Principle of Individual Work

John Adams says, "It is the most dramatic and systematic break away from the class teaching unit." In this method equal opportunities are provided to each student to work at his own speed and rate. In this method it is not essential that equal time is taken by each student but it aims at the achievement of a minimum uniform standard. According to Miss H. Parkurst, "It is a piece of machinery for putting into operation the principle of individual work."

(ii) The Principle of Freedom

In this method of teaching there are no arbitrary fixed periods, there are no classroom restrictions or rigidity or discipline. In the words of a scholar, "It aims at giving to the older child that freedom for self-development which has proved so valuable in the school life of the infant while at the same time ensuring that he shall master thoroughly the academic work required by the curriculum of the school."

(iii) The Principle of Self-Effort

In this method child gains knowledge through his own efforts.

(iv) The Principle of Co-operation

According to Miss H. Parkurst, "The school can only reflect the social experience of community when all its parts or groups develop the same intimate relations with one another as is found in society as a whole. The school should be organised in such a way as the pupils and teachers come in close interaction with one another." The students live and work together with the same teachers, in the same shared common workshops or laboratories.

(v) The Principle of Setting Goals

In this method a goal is set which provides a stimulus to the child to work in a way so as to attain the goal.

The Plan Work as Under

(i) *Assignments or Contracts:* After the teacher has outlined the work to be completed during a year, he divides and sub-divides it into various units and then be prepares the assignments. While preparing the assignments teacher keeps in mind various factors such as holidays, time available, revision at various stages, curriculum activities and the demand of other subjects.

Each subject has its separate assignment and the student must complete his first assignment in each subject before proceeding to a second assignment in any subject. Moreover, he must complete all the assignments for a particular period in time.

(ii) *Subject Teachers:* The student is guided and supervised by a subject teacher who is a specialist in his subject.

(iii) *Subject Rooms:* Each specialist is incharge of his subject room that is equipped with the material needed in that subject. The student is free to come to the room and devote as much time as he likes in a particular subject room.

(iv) *Records:* To show the work done by each student graphs are maintained. They serve as a mirror of pupil's work and also serve as a link between teacher and student. Such a graph is a contract remainder of the 'contract' or 'promise'.

(v) *Conference:* In after room session group discussions are arranged under the guidance of the teacher. Such discussions are known as 'conference' and these are devoted to remove common difficulties and also to explain certain items of common interest and importance.

Duties of a Teacher

Given below are some of the important duties of teacher in Dalton Plan:

(i) Preparation of assignments and giving them to the pupil as and when required.

(ii) Keeping an atmosphere of study in the room.

(iii) Giving explanations of any details of the assignment and removing the difficulties of the pupils.

(iv) Giving information with regard to the use of relevant equipment and materials.

(v) Ensuring the each assignment is finished properly before the new assignment is given to the pupil.

(vi) Keeping full records of the progress made by pupils in different classes.

(vii) Keeping the subject-library and other equipment up-to-date and in proper order.

The teacher, in the Dalton Plan, is "a helper, not a driver, the pursued, not the pursuer."

Merits of Plan

The plan has the following advantages:

(i) Individualised teaching.

(ii) Community of work.

(iii) Development of qualities such as self-effort and self-confidence.

(iv) Purposeful learning.

(v) Development of desirable study habits.
(vi) Development of a sense of responsibility.
(vii) Solving the problems of home-task.
(viii) Soving the problem of discipline.
(ix) Simplification of the problem of evaluation.
(x) Better pupils-teacher relationship.

Limitations of the Method

(i) Not suitable for the average child and a shirker.
(ii) Development of individualistic tendencies.
(iii) Purely intellectual plan.
(iv) Unsuitable for a lesson that needs inspiration treatment.
(v) Lack of suitable teachers.
(vi) Lack of well-equipped libraries.
(vii) Unsuitable for junior classes.
(viii) Very costly.
(ix) No provision for individual differences.

8. Discussion Method

Discussion is totally different from *debate*. In *debate* the participant makes an all-out effort to prove a point whereas in *discussion* the participants try to discover the truth. Discussion stimulates the mental activity and helps in developing fluency and ease in expression. An exchange of ideas and opinions offers valuable training to students in reflective thinking.

Important Constituents of Discussion.

Following are the important constituents:

(i) *The leader* — the teacher
(ii) *The group* — the class
(iii) *The problem* — the topics under discussion
(iv) *The content* — body of knowledge
(v) *Evaluation* — change in ideas, attitudes etc.

Directing Group Discussions

The teacher has to show immense patience and skill to ensure that discussion takes place on right lines and in the appropriate environment. Following points may be considered in this respect:

1. Students should be well-acquainted with the significance of the topic, its nature and scope and causes why the class should discuss it.
2. Discussion should be confined to important aspects.
3. Students should be encouraged to participate in the discussion.
4. Ideas may be invited without pressure or embarrassment.
5. Explanations, where needed, should be provided.
6. Personality cult should be avoided.
7. Co-operation rather than competition should be encouraged.
8. Efforts should be made to develop team spirit.
9. Doubts, mistakes and wrong interpretation should be made clear by the teacher.
10. Facts and points should be evaluated.
11. Facts and points should be summarised.
12. Students should be guided to honour difference of opinion and views.
13. Goals of discussions should be kept in view.
14. Only a few students should not be allowed to dominate class-room discussion.
15. Shy students may be given training in discussion in small groups so that their hesitation is removed while participating in bigger groups.

Organisation of Discussion

Following are the main techniques of organising a discussion:

1. Introducing a topic or a problem by the teacher by giving points or explanation to serve as the basis of discussion.
2. Calling upon a pupil by the teacher of give facts, describe a scence of situation, explain an incident, event of happening for getting the discussion started.

3. Preparing an outline of points co-operatively by the teacher and a few students which may become the starting point for discussion.
4. Asking the students to describe their own experiences connected with the subject, topic or problem and making them points for discussion.
5. Presenting detailed papers by the teacher and discussions thereon.
6. Presenting detailed papers by the students and discussing them in the class.
7. Showing special works and projects to the class and discussing them.
8. Showing some pictures charts, diagrams or any audiovisual material and discussion about them.

Merits of Discussion

1. It helps in clarifying issues.
2. It helps children in crystallizing their thinking.
3. It helps students in discovering what they do not know and what they have overlooked.
4. It engenders more reflection. It is farther from rote learning.
5. It represents a type of pooled knowledge, ideas and feelings of several persons.
6. It develops team spirit.
7. It engenders toleration of views which are at variance.
8. It affords opportunities to the students to learn together, make suggestions, share responsibility, comprehend the topic, evaluate the findings and to summarise results.
9. It provides opportunities to the students to speak distinctly, stand and sit correctly respect the ideas of others, share interests, ask pertinent questions and comprehend the problem before the group.
10. It helps the teacher in discovering talented students who have potential for becoming good leaders.

Limitations of Discussion

1. It is not suitable in all topics.
2. It is likely to be dominated by a few students.
3. It is likely to go off the track.
4. It may lead to unpleasant feelings.
5. It may create emotional tensions.
6. It may involve unnecessary arguments.

9. Problem Solving Method

In this method the student is required to solve a problem making use of his pervious knowledge. Problem solving may be defined as a planned attack upon a difficulty or perplexity in which a person makes use of his ability and capacity to find a suitable and satisfying solution. Yoakam and Simpson define it as, "A problem that occurs in a situation in which a felt difficulty is clearly present and recognised by the thinker. It may be purely mental difficulty or it may be physical and may involve manipulation of data. The distinguishing thing about a problem, however, is that an individual who meets it as needing a solution, recognising it as a 'challenge'. It is a method in which some difficulty of act in an educational setting is felt and an attempt is make is a conscious planned and purposeful way to find its solution."

Dewey observes, "whenever—no matter how slight and common place is character—a difficulty perplexes and challenges the mind so that it makes belief at all uncertain—there is a genuine problem." He further ties problem solving with reflective thinking as follows. "The problem fixes the end of thought and the end controls the process of thinking."

According to Gates, "A problem exists for an individual when he has a definite goal and he cannot reach by the behaviours patterns which he already available."

According to C.V. Good, "The problem method is a method of instructions by which learning is stimulated by the creation of challenging situations that demand solution. It is a specific procedure by which a major problem is solved through the combined solutions of a number of smaller problems."

Teachers who are problem-minded may consider the whole of the course of Social Studies as a big problem. Children like problems and feel interested in solving problems. Thus problem-solving can be used as a useful activity. However, success in problem solving depends upon how the problem is presented and how well is the child prepared to face it? Children will be able to solve problems successfully if we keep in mind the following characteristics of a good problem:

(i) The problems are of such nature that the students feel interested in them.

(ii) The problems are according to the age, need, mental and physical capacity and resourcefulness of pupils.

(iii) The problems are such as may provide the maximum of activity, and useful knowledge to pupils.

(iv) The problems are solved in original and cooperative atmosphere.

(v) The problems have educational values.

(vi) The problems are correlated with the physical and social environment of the pupils.

Thus the problem solving method is quite suitable for teaching of Social Studies in which we lay more emphasis on all the above mentioned points. The successful accomplishment of problem-solving is the goal towards which many other phases of the learning situation are directed. As distinguished from the Project Method, the Problem Method is characterised chiefly by mental activity, by critical thinking and is, therefore, more directly applicable to the secondary school level instruction. Just as the project method has better claim for excellence when used in the elementary school, the problem method produces good results when used with secondary school pupils.

General Principles of Problem Solving

1. ***The Pupils must feel the Problem their own:*** The problem must include interest plus values to arouse the curiosity of children for finding its solution, as it will fulfil their immediate need.
2. ***The Problem must be Stated Definitely:*** After the pupils have come to feel the problem as their own, the teacher

must see that it is stated in definite terms. If it is defined clearly, the pupils will be able to find out its solution without much difficulty.

3. ***Selecting Material for Problem Solving:*** The means of solving the problem must not be vague to the pupils. A judicious selection of the material must be made as it may be too vast and complicated in case of subjects like Social Studies, for secondary school students. Material must be according to the age and capacity of pupils. It should also be easily available.
4. ***Solutions must be Definite and Clear:*** Various means should be used to arrive at definite conclusions. One of the pupils should be asked to summarise the conclusion before the whole class. Then let the other pupils evaluate and criticise it until accepted by all. This definiteness of the conclusion or solution must be emphasised. The teacher, then, should help the pupils to apply the newly gained knowledge or skill to some immediate problem situation. The manner of application will depend upon the type of problem which has been solved. Thus problems become useful and educational and the matter pertaining to their solution also serves a useful purpose, if they are according to the base of reality, understanding and effect.

Steps in Problem-solving

Following are the important steps in problem-solving method:

(i) The formation and appreciation of the problem.
(ii) The collection of relevant data and material.
(iii) Organisation of data.
(iv) Drawing of conclusions.
(v) Testing conclusions.

Teacher's Role in Problem-solving Method

Quoting Professor Pasher, Valentine Deirs lists the following as role of the teacher in problem-solving method:

(i) To give the students a chance so that they define the problem clearly.

(ii) Help the students to keep the problem in mind.

(iii) Encourage the students to come forward with their suggestions. For this he should encourage them.

(a) to analyse the situations in parts;

(b) to recall previously known similar cases and general rules that apply;

(c) to guess and formulate guesses correctly.

(iv) Allow them time to evaluate the suggestions by encouraging them.

(a) to maintain a state of doubt a suspended conclusion;

(b) to criticise the suggestion by appeal to know facts, minister experiments and scientific treatises;

(v) Get them to organise material by proceeding

(a) to build an outline on the board;

(b) to use diagrams and graphs;

(c) to formulate concise statement of the net outcome of the discussion.

Advantages of the Problem Solving Method

1. ***It conforms to Life:*** Every one is confronted with problems all through life. Training in problem-solving, in the school, will help the pupils to form certain attitudes and skills, so essential for adult life. It, therefore, constitutes a realistic method for presenting the type of experience that will face the pupils throughout their career. They will be able to meet life situations with boldness, courage and success. Problem solving will prove to be a good preparation for solving personal and community difficulties in later life. by the pupils.
2. ***Develops the Power of Critical Judgement:*** Due to self-activity involved in problem solving pupils become interested in their study programme and develop the power of critical judgements. This is of vital importance in a democracy where the success of a government depends upon the judgement of the people.
3. ***It Makes for Pupils Activity:*** The pupils are stimulated to struggle for solutions of certain problems. They are, then,

no longer passive members of a class but active participants. They themselves make efforts to solve problems.

4. ***Knowledge Easily Assimilated:*** Knowledge is gained because of purposeful activity, connected with pupil's everyday life. So it is easily assimilated. It also remains permanently with the child because it has been gained in real life situation.
5. ***Develops the Traits of Open-mindedness and Tolerance:*** The pupils find that there are so many sides to a problem and they listen to different points of view. So they become tolerant in outlook and open-minded in their attitude. The attitude is very important in adult life these days.
6. ***It tends to Develop Initiative and Responsibility:*** The pupils begin to feel that the process is not a task which is assigned but an inevitable requirement of the situation. They, therefore, get a fine chance to think,-to judge and evaluate and to develop their initiative and responsibility. Such a development makes them useful and effective citizens in adult life.
7. ***It promotes Harmonious Relationship between the Teacher and Pupils:*** Teacher's guidance plays an important part in problem solving. The teacher has got the ability to see problems clearly the power to analyse with discernment and the facility to synthesise and draw conclusions with accuracy. So he is a rare help in the mastery of this difficult technique of problem-attack. The pupils soon learn to appreciate the guidance of the teacher in helping them to achieve their goal.

Limitations of this Method

1. ***Requires too much Reference Material:*** Some problems need too much reference material for their correct solution. All this material may not be available to students. Suitable books are also not available in the school library.
2. ***Takes too much Time:*** Preparation and initiation of the problem solving procedure may take a considerable portion of the teacher's time.Too much time of the class may also be consumed by this procedure. So it is not possible to make a continuous use of this method. The teacher has to cover

the vast syllabus in Social Studies, in each term, which may not be possible if he takes to teaching by this method. One problem may take weeks or even months for its solution. So this method is to be tried on certain occasions during the year, when the situation has actually been created for problem-solving.

3. ***Tends to Become Monotonous:*** If used too frequently it may become monotonous. If students continue working on one problem for days or weeks together, they lose interest in it. They want different types of activities on all occasions. If one and the same activity is continued for many days or weeks, it must become dull and uninteresting.
4. ***Does not always achieve Satisfactory Results:*** Satisfactory results may not be achieved due to certain factors. In that case the pupils may become dissatisfied and discouraged. They will feel that problem solving has been a sheer waste of time and energy. Such a feeling may develop wrong attitudes in them, like futility and cynicism etc.

Conclusion

Problem-solving is characteristic of reflective thinking. Modern methods claim provocation of thought as the main purpose of teaching. All educational procedures demand thinking on problem-solving. So this method can be used in all procedures or methods, which develop mental skills, attitudes and ideals.

9. Source Method

Source method implies the use of original material and original sources in teaching of Social Studies. Source can be classified as under:

(i) Primary source.

(ii) Secondary source.

The study and use of original sources, will give a much better understanding of subjects like Social Studies than any other method.

Original sources are of three kinds:

(i) *Material sources*, such as ruins, statues, tools, weapons, customs, traditions etc.

(ii) *Oral accounts*, such as songs, folk lores, anecdotes, customs, traditions etc.

(iii) *Written or printed records*, such as manuscripts, reports, diaries, letters, treaties, laws, newspapers, and account books etc.

In teaching of Social Studies we are mainly concerned with written and printed records.

Primary Source

They include physical remains or relics of unconscious testimony in far off historical sites, roads, pyramids, human remains, clothing, food, fortification, utensils, pottery, building, implements, machinery, furniture, weapons, fine arts and museum pieces, inscriptions etc.

They also include consciously transmitted information in the form of oral or written testimony. Such written sources are constitutions, charters, court decisions, official minutes or records, autobiographies, letters, diaries, genealogies, contracts, deeds, wills, permits, licences, affidavits, depositions, declarations, proclamations, certificates, bills, receipts, magazines and newspapers, accounts, advertisements, maps, diagrams, books pamphlets, films etc.

Secondary Source

These are the sources which are written by those who are not actually on the sense of the events, e.g., An act passed by the Parliament is a primary source but its extract published is a secondary source.

How to Utilise Sources?

The teacher can make use of sources in a variety of ways. Some of these are as follows:

(i) *Demonstration:* To convince the students about the utility of those sources the teacher should give a demonstration of the utilisation of these sources. For this he may read a passage from the original source, supporting or illustrating his point of view and throwing additional light on his opinion. In this way he will motivate his pupils to go through some such sources for clarifying certain controversial issues or for arriving at truth about a certain point. But the teacher should make it quite clear to his pupils that source material is to be employed at appropriate times rather than to be read for the sake of reading.

(ii) *Assigned Reading:* The teacher can use the sources by assigning selected passages to be read by students. However, he should see that all the selected passages should be interesting and immediately connected with the topic in hand.

(iii) *Problem Solving:* Problems can best be solved with the help of sources. The pupils will be able to discover and correct errors in the text-books and in other secondary accounts if any, with their help. The problem is to reach the truth and in this search, source method is of great help and advantage.

Difficulties in Utilizing Original Sources

There are, however, many difficulties in the utilisation of original sources. Some of them are as follows:

1. *Sources of real value not available:* In India original sources of real worth, suitable especially for school students, are too scanty and too disjoined. Efforts have not been made so far to edit and compile source books suitable for school students.
2. *Difficulty of language :* Almost all the original sources of historical or cultural value, are in language, foreign to Indian students. Our pupils in schools cannot be expected to deal with long passages in English, Sanskrit, Pali, Arabic or Persian, the languages in which most of the original sources are available. Relevant and short extracts from contemporary documents in the pupil's mother tongue can serve the desired purpose and these are seldom available.
3. *Conflicting views of different contemporary writers:* A source is not necessarily reliable merely because it is a source. Like all other writers, source writers also have their own prejudices, faults, preferences and limitations. Authors of different sources give different accounts of events or movements during the same period according to their own

points of view. The students are, thus lost in the maze of conflicting views about the same event or movement. They naturally feel that they cannot solve all the problems through the source method.

Use of Source Method

It can be used at following stages of the lesson:

1. *Pre-lesson use of resources.* Visits to actual sites of monuments, forts or museums may be arranged. The teacher can ask the students to read selected passages connected with the lesson before hand.
2. *Mid-lesson use of resources.* Extracts from original or secondary sources can be read during the course of the lesson. They create real situations, import reality and vividness to the lesson and reinforce the impact of teaching.
3. *Post-lesson use of resources.* Pre-lesson use of resources can also become the post-lesson use of resources and vice-versa. Students may be given assignments which need use of resources. They may be encouraged to pursue their interest in a particular topic, do some critical thinking and analysis and prepare their own account.

Advantages of the Source Method

The following advantages may be derived occasionally by following the source method:

1. It would make facts appear real, as they are gathered from sources which can be seen or studied directly. The learner acquires greater conviction in regard to the truth of happenings.
2. The source method provides an opportunity to the pupils to learn civics and political science by 'doing'. It is activity method. The activities may take very interesting shape in the form of visits to museums, actual handling of things in the school museum, etc.
3. The source method offers scope for groups work— there may be a workshop for building up history in regard to a particular topic with the help of sources.

4. This method gives the pupils an insight into the process of gathering facts and it develops the historical sense in them. The sense of objectivity which is very important to a student of social studies and political science can be particularly developed through this method.
5. This method also gives the pupils some idea about the method of historical research, however rudimentary the idea might be. As such this method may make some contribution in developing the interest of pupils in research though they may undertake it at a much later date.
6. Though the source method may be more suitable to the pupils of higher classes, it can also be utilised with advantage by pupils of primary classes, who may, be studying political science and civics through the source method. The source method would make their study more concrete and more meaningful.
7. It supplements classroom lesson.
8. It develops elementary skills of collecting data sifting the relevant and organising the same.
9. Learning becomes functional because it is gained in the real situation.
10. It provides opportunities for useful mental exercises — right thinking and imagining, comparing and analysing drawing inferences, etc.

Steps to be Followed in Source Method

The steps, to be followed in studying a topic through the source method are as under:

(i) The unit for study, with problems and source materials through which answers are to be sought, should first be presented to the pupils. Reference in regard to the source material may also be given to the pupils.

(ii) If we wish to follow the workshop technique, the class should be divided into groups with assignment of specific responsibilities, i.e. each group should be given a few specific questions whose answers it may try to find out with the help of source materials.

(iii) After this the pupils should be introduced to the sources (excursions to sites, visits to museums and the student or group should seek the solution of the problems assigned to them (the group may make its own sub-division of responsibilities among its members).

(iv) One or two class periods may then be provided to the groups for editing the notes (taken while in direct contact with the sources) and for preparing written answers to the questions assigned to them.

(v) The answers may be mutually corrected by the group according to the procedure suggested before; the teacher may also go through the answers, select the best ones and keep them in a convenient place for use by the pupils.

(vi) One class period (if it can be spared) may be devoted to the discussion of some of the controversial findings arrived at by the groups, with a view to stimulate greater interest in the work.

(vii) The groups may also be encouraged to write articles for the social studies wall newspaper on the basis of their findings.

Limitations of the Source Method

1. It is very difficult for the school teachers to have an easy access to original sources.
2. Utilisation of original sources is a very difficult task for the school students as they lack the requisite training.
3. The method is very complex and technical.
4. There is the difficulty of languages. Almost all the original sources are in the Sanskrit, Pali, Arabic or Persian and a few in English.
5. Contemporary authors and writers have given their own prejudices, preferences and limitation with the result that it becomes very difficult to sift fact from fiction. The students are, thus, lost in the maze of conflicting view about the same event or movement.
6. Source method of teaching is very expensive.
7. Source method of teaching is time consuming.

How to Make Source Method Effective?

The students be encouraged to study the resource books in the library. Educational tours to places of importance may be arranged. The students may be asked to write their own impressions and inferences about the places they visit. Copies of important extracts from the relevant records may be pasted on the blackboard for the use of students.

Dr. Keatings thinks that original sources can be used for creating suitable environment in the lower form. Well-planned, purposive and well-directed efforts have to be made by the teacher in the use of this method. By suggesting the use of resource method we do not aim at making our students research scholars. Use of the method in selected topics is likely to make the study of political science and social studies meaningful and real.

10. Recitation or Socialised Recitation Method

Adam Wesley was one of the chief exponents of this method. He wanted to introduce a method in which the whole class acquires knowledge with the co-operation of all the students. In this method of the formal character of the classroom is intended to be dismantled. The students are encouraged to acquire knowledge according to their nature, interest and the co-operation of their fellow beings. In this method the students are asked to sit in the classroom in a semi-circle. The teacher takes his seat alongwith the students. This method is also known as 'Socialised Discussion Method'.

According to Harold Benjamin, the following are the main purposes of Socialised Recitation:

(i) to develop technique useful to group work;
(ii) to stimulate reflective thinking;
(iii) to supplement previous knowledge;
(iv) to encourage creative expression.
(v) to develop desirable social attitudes by providing practice in a large variety of specialised situations;
(vi) to practise in the technique of cooperative thinking;

In the olden times, there were many defects in recitation. The major defect was that it laid more emphasis on teacher activity to the neglect of pupil activity.

The subject-matter occupied the most important place in teaching. The drilling of the fact into the minds of the pupils was considered to be the main function of teacher. Naturally, under such a procedure, the pupils felt indifferent, lifeless and dull. To motivate study under these conditions was almost an impossibility. The pupils regarded their lesson as a tedious and tiresome task.

It was suggested that emphasis must be taken from the teacher and placed on the pupils. The old system of teaching must be replaced by a new procedure of Socialized Recitation. This procedure brought about more pupil activity and a liberation of school control. It brought a new era in the class-room which made the pupil and his activities more prominent than the teacher or the subject-matter. Group discussions have become very common. Text-book is supplemented by various devices and aids of teaching. Under such conditions the pupil's personality develops in a natural way. Incentive is provided for exercising initiative, originality and independent thinking. Group thinking is developed and class-room becomes a unit of dynamic group life. An atmosphere of freedom and naturalness prevails. The traditional class is transformed into a socialized one which is not dominated by a few individuals but belongs to all members of the class. In fact "Group consciousness and the feeling of individual responsibility towards the group" is a Socialized Recitation.

How to Proceed in Socialized Recitation

Informal Socialized Recitation is not rigidly organised. It may assume any form, from a simple informal organisation to a complex parliamentary one. It can be a sort of committee meeting in which the members decide on an agenda, express their ideas freely, share their information willingly and come to some definite conclusions about a certain issue or problem. The discussion may be carried on by the class as a whole with the teacher, acting as leader of the discussion. It may be only a form of socialized group discussion in which members of the group elect their own chairman to guide the discussion. It may also have a president, a secretary and other elected officials and carry out the discussion in a parliamentary procedure. It should, however, be remembered that no procedure can be used exactly the same way by all teachers. Both teachers and classes have different characteristics. A wise teacher should evaluate these forms and use them in building up a technique of his own.

A general plan of socialized procedure that has been used with success in many schools is one in which the lesson or topic is divided into four or five parts. The class is also divided into four or five groups. Each group of students, under its own chosen student leader, is assigned one part of the lesson. Each group then plans its own work and executes it according to its own plan. All this planning however, is to be approved by the teacher, though he does not dictate things during the lesson. In groups, questions are asked, comments are offered and discussions are held freely and frankly. The members of the group are free to discuss any point that has not been made clear to them. After the group has completed the discussion, the leader will offer additional information that he thinks essential. Then all the groups will meet together to place their observations and conclusions before the whole class. The teacher will, then, offer his own remarks if he feels that certain points have not been touched upon by the pupils or if definite conclusions have not been reached. In order to provide equal opportunities to all pupils, the leadership should be changed from lesson to lesson. This will infuse confidence even in those students who are considered to be intellectually backward.

Role of the Teacher

The success of this procedure will, depend upon the role, the teacher plays throughout. He is to set the stage, give the promptings as and when necessary and then sum up the conclusions or generalisations, arrived at. All this work is not easy. Socialized Recitation will succeed with the careful planning and judicious guidance of the teacher. But the teacher no longer dominates the scene. He is simply a member of group. He retains control of the class but as a guide, a leader, an adviser and a helper rather than a traditional master.

Merits or Advantage

This method of teaching has certain advantages in it.

(i) It trains the students in the art of making plans and encourages them to take up work independently. The students are also asked to take part in the discussions and debates. They are encouraged to take up independent thinking.

(ii) The students are trained in organising their experience and put them down in a written form.

(iii) This method tries to discover the interest and aptitudes of the students.

(iv) This method is helpful in creating self-confidence and self-reliance in the students.

This method requires a very careful handling. Teacher shall have to be trained before this method can be put to practice. That training programme is yet to be achieved.

Disadvantages of Socialized Recitation

1. *Inadequate mastery of the subject-matter:* From the point of view of the acquisition and mastery of subject-matter, the use of this method is not at all desirable. Many other procedures, are much more efficient and useful in this respect. Much more time is uselessly wasted if we follow Socialized Recitation procedure and time, at our disposal, is limited. The importance of this method lies only in the social values involved.

2. *Tendency to wander away from the topic:* Another great drawback of this method is the tendency of the class to wander away from the subject proper. Therefore, careful guidance is essential on the part of the teacher. He must be able to lead the class to the point at issue through his tact and resourcefulness. He cannot be merely a stage-setter and a passive spectator of the lesson.

3. *Danger of futile discussion:* The recitation may lead to futile discussion. Some students are in the habit of arguing things for the sake of argument alone. Others may argue simply to prove their point, whether it has any direct connection with the lesson and topic in hand or not. On such occasions the teacher should be alert enough to prevent useless debates.

4. *Danger of domination by a few assertive pupils:* In this procedure there is always the danger that a few pupils may

dominate the entire lesson. Such domination is not conducive to the full values that should result from the use of this method. It is, therefore, the duty of the teacher to plan recitation in such a way that the lesson is not monopolised by a few students. The teacher must be interested in the socialization of all the pupils and not merely a few of them.

5. *Danger in the exclusive use of Socialized Recitation:* Some champions of modern procedures, recommended the exclusive use of this method at all times. This is a dangerous move. As we have already noted, there are times to use this method and times when it is not to be used at all. As far as socialization itself is concerned, it is highly desirable that every lesson should more or less be socialized in the sense that students are given chances to participate actively in it. But mere socialization cannot serve the purpose in case of a vast subject like Social Studies.

Conclusion

Socialized Recitation may prove very useful if used with other methods and procedures. It may be profitably used for review-work and for problem-solving. It may also be associated with supervised study. This combination with other procedures can be used very successfully in the class-room. Moreover, the socialized procedure can make use of all the devices, projects, problems and activities which are available under other methods.

As in the case of all other methods, we should not think that Socialized Recitation is a solution to all class-room problems. It is only a procedure which may frequently be used by the teacher to much advantage. But teaching is not a mechanical process and as such no ONE method can be recommended for all occasions. Success in the use of Socialized Recitation will depend upon the class, the teacher and the aim of the lesson that teacher keeps before him.

11. Survey Method

In this method, the students are encouraged to discover and survey things and thereby acquire knowledge. In this, the students are encouraged to survey the local conditions and environments. This method is useful for lower classes. Here the whole class is divided into various groups and each group is asked to survey a particular aspect of a subject. For example, a class may be divided into five groups--one group may be asked to survey the geographical conditions of the city, another group may be asked to survey the history of the origin and the development of the city. The third group may be asked to collect the data about to the number of shops in the city, the fourth group may be asked to collect information about occupations and local administration and other social problems.

When the students have made a survey of the fields allocated to them, they collect together and discuss them and arrive at a certain conclusion. Then they write out the conclusions in systematic manner. Maps and graphs are also drawn. These maps and charts are used for decorating the walls of the classroom.

In fact, this method of teaching is nothing but a combination of various methods. It has the element of a scientific procedure of study.

12. Dramatic Method or Play Method

This method is based on the theory of 'Play'. Attempt is made to get the subject-matter enacted or dramatised with the help of the students. The students take interest in dramatising the subject-matter. While dramatising, they acquire knowledge.

This is a psychological method. The students remain active in the acquisition of knowledge.

In this method of teaching the working of the Parliament or Zila Parishads may be dramatised with the help of the students.

This method is also likely to develop the creative efforts of the educands.

Merits of the Dramatic Method

It has the following merits in it:

1. It brings about a development of the mental faculties of the students.
2. Through this method, interest is created in the students about the subject that has to be taught.
3. Through this method the subject-matter of Social Studies is made interesting and intelligible.

4. This method creates in the students, a sense of self-confidence and self-importance. Shyness of the students is dismantled.
5. It also leads to development of social and moral qualities in the students. They try to live up to the ideals of the great men whose role they play.

Requirements

This method requires certain things from the teacher:

1. The teacher should be well-aware of the techniques of drama. He should also know the art of writing dialogues.
2. He should have the capacity to select the dramatic material.
3. He should also be acquainted with the qualities of simplicity and authenticity that are requisites of dramatic procedure.
4. The teacher should have the capacity to mould his personality accordingly as and when required. In short, he should have all that practical knowledge that is required for an efficient Drama Director.

13. Comparative Method

This method was propounded by the famous educationist, Aristotle. He was of the view the Social Studies is a subject which is a combination of many subjects. These subjects are similar as well as different. The teacher should, therefore, try to teach the subject of Social Studies on the basis of various methods. He should try to compare various things and thus impart knowledge of the Social Studies to the students. While resorting to comparative method, following things should be borne in mind:

1. Conclusion should be arrived at only after comparing various things. It is not wise to compare two things only and then jump down to a conclusion.
2. Comparison should always be done with the similar things. If the comparison is to be made of certain associations, various social, cultural, political and other associations should be taken up and they should be compared from various angles.

14. Narration Method or Method of Narration or Story Method

In this method, the teacher narrates the subject-matter before the students. He tries to explain the indirect knowledge through his direct narration. An attempt is made to present the difficult subject-matter in a simple, intelligible and interesting manner. If this method is combined by question-answer method, it becomes all the more interesting. But it is not possible to employ this method in the teaching of each and every subject. The teacher should handle this method cautiously. He should not dominate the whole scene. He should also encourage the students to remain active.

This method may be quite useful in the teaching of Social Studies. Certain topics may be taught in a narrative method. The teacher should keep the following things in view:

1. In narration, the age, interest and the aptitude of the child should be borne in mind. The narration should be clear, systematic, interesting and well-organised. There should be perfect chronological order.
2. The narration should have the element of administration in it. The teacher should show certain pictures etc. to the students.
3. The voice of the teacher should be quite attractive. He should have the capacity to change his voice according to emotions and circumstances. His pronunciation should be very clear and scientific.

The following statement of Binings in regard to the method of teaching is quite important:

> "If the teaching is to reach its highest degree of efficiency, teacher must possess a broad understanding of all faces of method as a part of that Philosophy of Education which is essential to good teaching."

REVISION QUESTIONS

1. Describe text-book method of teaching Social Studies.
2. What is problem method? What is the role of teacher in problem method?
3. What are various methods of teaching of Social Studies?

Which method is useful for which stage of education?

4. What is the importance of method in the teaching-learning process?
5. What part does the personality of the teacher play in method?
6. Show the difference between a project method and problem method of teaching.

6

Audio Visual Aids in Social Studies

6.1 INTRODUCTION

In Social Studies we are concerned with the study of man and his relationship with his environment. In order to understand it we need a rich background. This background is provided through a large variety of sight and sound experiences. Experiences are the individual's reactions to life situations as they occur. The teacher tries to teach social behaviour and relationship by providing desirable experiences.

According to estimates of Joseph J. Weber, nearly 40% of our concepts are based on visual experiences, 25% on auditory, 17% on the sense of touch and feeling, 15% upon miscellaneous organic sensation and 3% upon taste and smell.

As senses are the gateway of learning, we should try to provide the pupils with as many of sensory experiences as are possible. The teacher should integrate the use of various devices and must select that device which is likely to prove most effective in a given situation. While making his selection teacher should give due consideration to the age, sex, intelligence, experience of his pupils. He should make an effort to widen the scope of learning beyond the immediate environment of the child.

6.2 WHAT IS AN AUDIO-VISUAL AID?

Audio-visual aid is, "any device which by sight or sound increases the individual's experience, beyond that acquired through reading."

An audio-visual aid is only a means of stimulating interest at a particular time, during the course of a lesson and aids are not the ends but only additional means to particular ends. An aid must provoke an additional mental activity, it must satisfy a felt need and improve the pupil's understanding about that particular topic for which it has been utilized. The teaching aids must supplement the process of learning and should be used in full context to some point in the lesson. The aids must not be used merely for their entertainment value.

6.3 IMPORTANCE OF AUDIO-VISUAL AIDS

At present the education is child centred and no more subject-centred. Thus it is the aptitude, interest and mental powers of the children that determine the education. The aim of education is to develop and train the mental powers of the child. Teaching aids are used to make the teaching interesting.

If the education fails to create activity in the children or to awaken their interest in the subject-matter it is useless. For awakening interest the education should be practical and good.

We should make an effort to make the knowledge stable and strengthen the experiences. The method used for imparting education must be simple, interesting and intelligible. For this teacher has to make use of different methods, these methods must be such as to conform to the mental and psychological requirements of the child.

Teaching aids are the various things that bring about a better method and a system of education. They add to the effectiveness and attractiveness of the teaching.

About teaching aids Bining and Bining has said:

> "Visual devices of many kinds may serve in making the abstract concrete and in arousing interest in students that would otherwise be unreal and dull."

In the words of Edgar Bruce Wesely, "Audio-visual aids furnish experiences. This facilitates the association of objects and words. They save pupils, time and they provide simple and authentic information. They enrich and extend one's appreciation and furnish pleasant entertainment. They provide a simplified view of a complicated data. They stimulate the imagination and develop the pupil's power of observation. These aids may need explanation but they do not need translators. They speak a universal language of form, colour, position and motion. They constitute one of the royal roads to learning." If these aids are used properly after careful consideration, they will give many advantages. Some of the advantages of the use of teaching aids are given in succeeding section.

Importance of Teaching Aids

(i) They make the lesson of history interesting.

(ii) They help to stabilize the knowledge of the subject.

(iii) They make the process of learning interesting and practical.

(iv) They help the teacher to proceed 'from concrete to abstract'.

(v) They help the teacher to conduct the teaching efficiently and creditably.

(vi) They are a good substitutes for direct experiences and are a supplement to direct experience.

(vii) They are very helpful for poor readers and slow-learners.

(viii) They help to develop the power of imagination and observation.

(ix) They provide an opportunity for a change in the monotonous atmosphere that generally prevails in the class-room.

(x) They provide an opportunity for a better rapport between the teacher and his pupil.

(xi) They help the pupil to develop a scientific attitude.

(xii) They provide a training in scientific method.

(xiii) They can be used in bigger classes.

(xiv) Use of such aids is based on the principles of psychology.

6.4 NEED OF TEACHING AIDS

(i) These aids help the teacher getting the attention of his students.

(ii) These aids help in creating the interest of the student in the topic and activate the mental process of the students.

(iii) The student gets an opportunity to get a first hand experience by visualising some concrete things, living specimens and actual demonstrations etc.

(iv) Use of teaching aids help to have a clear conception of ideas, information, facts and principles.

(v) It helps the students in understanding some complicated and difficult concepts.

(vi) They provide an opportunity for a change in the monotonous atmosphere that generally prevails in a classroom.

(vii) They provide an opportunity for a better support between the teacher and his pupil.

(viii) They help the students to develop a scientific attitude.

(ix) They provide a training in scientific method.

(x) They can be used in bigger classes.

(xi) Use of such aids is based on the principles of psychology.

6.5 PRINCIPLES FOR USE OF TEACHING AIDS

Teaching aids should be used properly to make teaching more effective. Teaching can become more effective if such aids are used widely but the use of such aids cannot provide a guarantee of good teaching. Following points are important for use of teaching aids:

(i) Teaching aids should be woven with class-room teaching and these aids should be used only to supplement the oral and written being done in the class.

(ii) While making use of any teaching aid an effort be made that the teaching aids being used in any class are in conformity with the intellectual level of the students and is in accordance with the previous experience of the students.

(iii) Only such aids be preferred which provide a stimulus to the students for greater thinking and activity.

(iv) If possible actual specimens be preferred to a photograph or a slide of a specimen.

(v) The teaching aid used should be exact, accurate and real as far as practicable.

(vi) The teacher should use a teaching aid only when he is quite sure about handling a specific teaching aid. For handling some aids (e.g., operating a projector etc.) training is provided by various authorities. For this purpose more information can be obtained from local SCERT or directly from NCERT, New Delhi.

(vii) Teaching aids used be such as are closely related to pupil's experiences.

(viii) The teacher should use a teaching aid only after a proper planning so that the aid is used exactly at the point; in the process of teaching, where it best fits in the process of teaching.

(ix) Teacher should see that a follow up programme follows the lesson wherein a teaching aid has been used.

(x) Teacher should carry out occasional evaluation about the use, function and effect of a teaching aid on the learning process.

6.6 TYPES OF TEACHING AIDS

For convenience of discussion the teacing aids in social studies may be grouped as under:

(i) Aids used in elementary schools.

(ii) Aids used in secondary schools.

As a matter of fact no clear cut demarcation is possible but this categorisation is done only for convenience of study. The aids used in elementary schools may be called *elementary aids* and those more commonly used in secondary schools are referred to *aids useful for secondary schools.*

Materials used in the teaching of social studies are of the following kinds:

(i) *Traditional aids*: These included test-books, black-boards etc.

(ii) *Visual aids*: Objects, models, pictures, charts, sketch, map etc.

(iii) *Audio-visual aids*: Radio, film strip, tape-recorder, slide projector, television etc.

6.7 MATERIAL AIDS IN TEACHING OF SOCIAL STUDIES AT THE PRIMARY STAGE OF EDUCATION

At this stage of education, children between 6 to 11 years of age receive education. Their social, moral, mental and physical education does not take place simultaneously and at the same speed. It differs from child to child. As the children grow, their physical and mental organs find development. Therefore, it is not possible to employ one set of teaching aids on all the students simultaneously. It should differ from stage to stage.

Primary education is the stage of early childhood of the students: Students are very fond of listening to stories. Curiosity is their predominant instinct. The teacher should make an effort to impart education by playing upon this instinct of the children. Education should be of concrete nature.

An attempt also should be made to make the teaching interesting and attractive. Different types of teaching aids should be used but the consideration of the mental and the physical age group of the children should also be held in mind.

Text-books: At this stage children should not be taught with the help of text-books. However, the text-books may be used only for helping the students to revise and strengthen the experiences given to them in the classroom. The text-books that are used should be well-illustrated, attractive and nicely printed.

Models: At this stage of education generally Panchayats, Zila Parishads etc., are taught. Models of these things may be presented before the students. These models should be attractive and artistic. Students should be encouraged to prepare such models. This shall encourage their learning by doing.

Pictures and Charts: Pictures should be freely used at this stage of education. Showing of pictures satisfy the curiosity of the students. But while using these pictures, it should be borne in mind that they should be accurate, artistic and attractive.

To understand the physical and social activities of man in the background of his physical and natural environments pictures are quite useful. They give two dimensional representation to historical phenomenon and help in making history real. Besides presenting portraits of great personalities, pictures may be conveniently utilized to represent men and ideas. They can be used to represent the essential facts of history/social studies.

Qualities of a Good Picture

(i) It should be accurate and truthful.
(ii) It should possess illuminating captions.
(iii) Pictures of scenes should have comments of the author or the teacher.
(iv) It should be simple.
(v) It should be of some appropriate size.

In recent years with tremendous developments in the field of science and technology, with the help of projectors, the teacher can create the third dimension illusion, sustain the interest of the pupils in the topic and enable them to understand the past happening in their true setting.

Various types of pictures in use are:

(a) *Still pictures*: These are projected with the help of opaque projectors, film strip projector, magic lantern etc.
(b) *Motion pictures*: They represent historical events in their proper perspective, showing their casual sequence and continuity. The emotional impact of such films is enormous and historical facts and events are remembered easily.
(c) *Films*: There are various types of films such as (i) Class-room films, (ii) Documentary films etc. These films can bring into class-room such as element of realism which cannot be attained by any other medium of instruction.
(d) *Film strips or Film slides*: These are easy and simple to use. Many a film strips covering various parts of history are available. These are quite helpful to give the students useful knowledge of Social Studies in an interesting way.

Regarding films the remarks of great scientist Edison are, "The only text-book needed will be for the teacher's own use. Films will serve as guide posts to these teacher instruction books and not the books as guide to the films. Pupils will learn from films every thing that is there in every grade from the lowest to the highest. Films are inevitable as practically the sole teaching method."

Slow motion film is very useful from instruction point of view because it makes such process visible as cannot be seen by the naked eye. But it is not possible in case of motion picture to skip over some scenes and to devote more attention to some and less to others. It is not possible to change the sequence either as can be done in case of strips and slides.

How to Select and Use Films in Social Studies

To get maximum benefits out of films they should be carefully selected by the teacher. For selection of films teacher should keep in mind the following guidelines:

(i) The films should be relevant to the main idea of the unit of study or the topic under discussion.

(ii) It should develop concepts, aspects of human behaviour and other learning appropriate to the group.

(iii) It should be suitable for the pupils for whom it is to be used.

(iv) It should improve skills and expressions.

(v) It must be accompanied by a follow up programme.

Source of Films

Some important sources of films are:

1. The departments of education in Universities,
2. Ministry of Broadcasting and Ministry of Education,
3. Foreign embassies,
4. Extension service department and audio-visual departments of states.

They consist of a series of still pictures, printed on strips of motion picture film. Each of the individual film is known as a frame. Film strips come either in a single or a double frame. They vary in length from about one to four foot. Since they are cheap, schools can maintain their own library of film strips. They are quite easy to catalogue and store.

Advantages of Film Strips

(i) It can serve as a good readiness for map reading.

(ii) It can be used to show physical features of different states of India.

(iii) They can be used to introduce children to other countries of the world.

(iv) They can be used to show developmental features.

(v) They can be used to exhibit the growth and development of an area.

(vi) They can be used to introduce a unit.

(vii) They can be used for explanation and clarification.

(viii) They can be used for summary of lesson.

(ix) They can be used to emphasize certain points.

Charts

The charts are very useful teaching aids because they help the teacher to explain the point which otherwise would be difficult to explain. The charts help in creating a suitable subject atmosphere in the class-room and in elucidating various points. Charts help in saving time because instead of drawing them on the black-board, the teacher can depend upon the pre-drawn diagram on black-board with accuracy.

It is better if the charts of the topic being dealt with in the class are depicted prominently in fairly good numbers. Charts should be changed with the topic.

Use of Charts

In teaching of Social Studies there is a lot of scope for the use of charts. With the help of charts things can be presented in their usual form. In lower classes pictures are more useful where as in higher classes charts are considered better. Charts are used to explain relationships of various objects. They can present an outline of certain facts in useful manner.

Suggestions for Effective Use of Charts

Following points should be kept in mind while using charts as teaching aids:

(i) The chart should be neatly prepared. Important results or figures should be systematically drawn.

(ii) The size of a diagram, figure or shape should be appropriate. It should neither be too big nor too small.

(iii) To draw attention to some specific points different colours can be used while making a chart.

(iv) Charts should be accurate.

(v) The charts or a portion of the chart be depicted only for a short duration whenever it is needed.

(vi) It is desirable that the students are encouraged to prepare simple charts.

Precautions in Regard to Use of Charts

1. Charts should be simple and relevant to topic.
2. They should be apt for the standard of education at which they are being used.
3. They should be natural and artistically drawn.
4. In lower classes the charts should be rarely used, however in higher classes they should be used as and when required.

Examples of Charts

1. *How Glaciers change our land surface.*

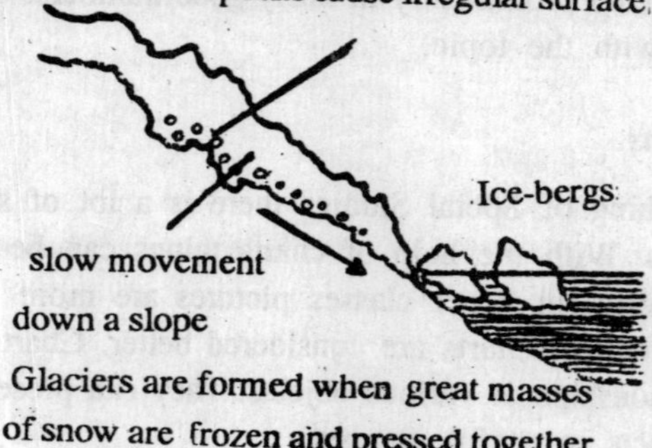

2. *Why the Season?*

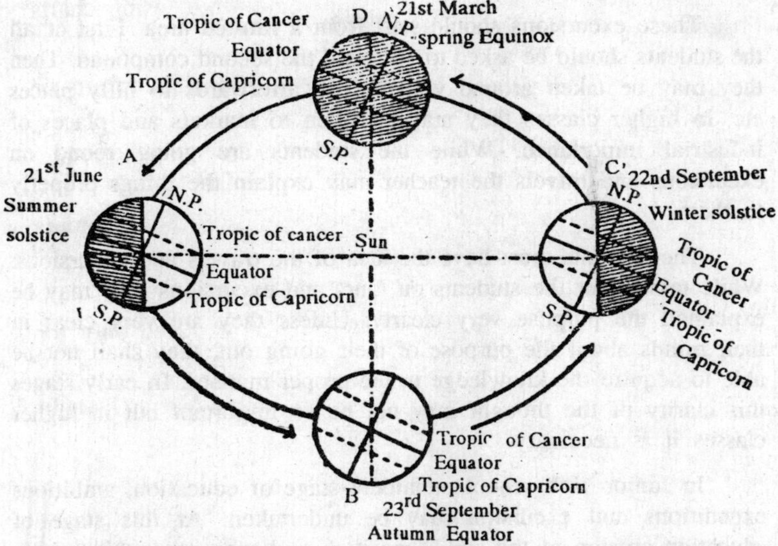

Other Audio-visual Aids for teaching to Social Studies at the secondary stage are:

1. Field Trips and Excursions

Excursions and trips provide an opportunity for the direct study of original materials in history. Visits to places of worship, tombs etc., help to break the monotony of class-room lectures and provide a chance to come in direct contact with historical realities. These are the most important and most effective devices of teaching social studies. A visit to a factory, a will, an irrigation project, a dam, a hospital, a post-office, a town hall, an assembly hall, a police station, a bank, a sea port, a museum, a zoo, a church, a temple, a mosque, a gurdwara, a visit to a hotel, a studio, a court, an airport etc., provide the students a first hand knowledge of different amenities of modern life.

The students may be taken to places of agriculture and industrial importance and there they may be made acquainted with various problems of industry and production.

Beginning from Limited Area and Going to Vaster Fields

These excursions should start from a limited area. First of all the students should be asked to go round the second compound. Then they may be taken around villages and afterwards to hilly places etc. In higher classes they may be taken to markets and places of industrial importance. While the students are going round on excursions and travels the teacher may explain the things properly to them.

The students must have the idea of the travels and excursions. While taking out the students on tours and excursions they may be explained the purpose very clearly. Unless they are very clear in their minds about the purpose of their going out, they shall not be able to acquire the knowledge in the proper manner. In early stages this clarity of the thought may not be so important but in higher classes it is necessary.

In Junior high school or middle stage of education, ambitious expeditions and excursion may be undertaken. At this stage of education erosion of the soil, deposition and such other things may be taught.

After the excursion the students be asked to write out what they have seen. This would strengthen their knowledge and experience. They may also be asked to draw models, charts, pictures, etc.

In higher classes the students may be taken out to places of industrial and agricultural importance. Such places can provide knowledge to the students. After coming back from the travels and excursions the students should be asked and encouraged to write down what they have seen.

The Requisites of Travels and Excursions

While taking out the students for travels and excursions the teacher should keep the following points in mind:

1. Discipline should be maintained while the students are going out. It can be done easily if the teacher continues to direct students properly and provide them an opportunity to see things in the proper perspective. If the students get interested in their observation they shall not be indisciplined.

2. While the students are being taken out to excursions they be made comfortable. For this they should be lodged properly and given proper food. If the students are not physically comfortable their mind shall not work properly and it shall not be possible for them to acquire knowledge in proper manner.
3. The teacher should direct the students in proper manner. He should explain the importance of each and everything that the students have seen. He may also explain which things are used for map drawing and which things are useful for charts.
4. After the excursions or travels the teacher should point out the particular chapter that may have bearing on the excursion or the travel. Such a reading will strengthen the experience and give a solid foundation to the knowledge.
5. Students should invariably be asked and encouraged to carry a note-book with them while they go out on excursions. They should also be encouraged to note down important things. Such things shall be useful in the class-room and proper study of the subject.
6. While an excursion the students should be encouraged to collect things that are of economical importance.

Dr. Heidgerken has summed up the **advantage of field trips** as an aid, in the following words:

(i) They furnish first hand information to supplement and enrich class-room instruction.

(ii) They correlate and blend school life with the outside world, providing direct touch with persons with community situations.

(iii) They create situations which help to develop observation and keenness. Field trips also offer an opportunity to apply that which has been taught and to verify what has been learned.

(iv) They provide actual source material for study.

(v) They arouse interest and vitalise instructions, thereby providing motivation.

(vi) They came as effective means of supplementing the subjects of the curriculum.

(vii) They necessitate planning, co-operation, security of transportation and permission to take the trip and other details of organisation. Thus they give training in shouldering and discharging responsibility to both pupils and teachers.

Thus we can say that, "definite planning, study, discussion, preparation, follow up and evaluation are essential if the full value and objectives of field trips are to be achieved."

2. Text-books

Text-books have been in vogue since times immemorial. These text-books are collection of facts and the knowledge about the subject-matter. Text-books have become quite popular since the invention of printing press.

Text-books give continuity and cohesion to the teaching process. A well chosen text-book forms useful basis in new lesson and affords material for home-task. In use of text-books teachers should take extra precaution to select only modern and recent text-book and reference book.

In the present educational setup the role of text-book is of prime importance. However, we find that a little attention is paid to this important aspect of education. Most of the text-books in Economics are not of good standard. They follow the prescribed syllabus too rigidly and no attention is paid to develop topics according to the need and interest of the students. A good text-book is one which is a source of knowledge arranged systematically. It enables the teacher to acquire the needed information quickly. It inspires the student to invent, to discover and to inculcate scientific methods. However, teacher should not depend solely as the best of the text-books because even such a text-book omits many details which teacher wants to tell to his students.

The use of the text-book is made by the students for completing the preparatory part of an assignment. They also use their text-books for doing revision of course. Some students also consult and use text-books to study at home. In this way the text-books are used to supplement the class-work. Text-books also provide a help to students in correct understanding of basic concepts and principles of social studies.

Generally a number of books are prescribed by board or university to be used as text-books. NCERT prepared text-books are available upto class XII. While recommending a text-book to his students the teacher should consider the following points to assess the worth of the book.

(i) Correctness of matter.

(ii) Purity of language.

(iii) Simplicity of diagrams.

(iv) Quality of printing and binding.

(i) Correctness of Matter

In this connection the standing of the author and the reputation of the publishers should be considered. The books written by well-known author having a long teaching experience of teaching the subject and possessing requisite qualifications be recommended. It would be much appreciated if certain minimum qualification and experience for authors is laid by authorities.

(ii) Purity of Language

A text-book that presents the subject-matter in a simple, clear and lucid language should be preferred. For text-books in a regional language, the terminology should also be given in English within brackets. In such books only standard terminology evolved by the Central Ministry of Education and State Governments should be used.

(iii) Simplicity of Diagrams

Only simple and well-labelled diagrams be given in text-books. Such diagrams are self-explanatory and help the students in properly understanding the subject-matter.

(iv) Quality of Printing and Binding

It is desirable that a text-book makes use of good quality paper and the quality of printing, and type letters is fine. It should be bound that its binding is appealing to the students.

In addition to the above a good text-book is expected to select and arrange the subject-matter in a psychological sequence. The book should follow the aim of teaching social studies. Each chapter start with a brief introduction and a summary of subject-matter be given at the end of each chapter. Some assignments should also be given at the end of each chapter and the assignments should cover such areas as applicable to life situations. Headings and sub-headings be given in bold type. A table of contents be provided at the beginning and a subject index be provided at the end. Glossary of some important terms be given at the end of the book.

While evaluating a book the teacher should apply objective tests like the following:

1. The contents should be accurate and adequate for the age level and should conform with the syllabus.
2. The concept should not be difficult or ambiguous.
3. The literary style should encourage the students to read the text-book and the vocabulary should be well-chosen.
4. Photographs should be well-produced.
5. The quantity and quality of illustration should be reasonably good.
6. The general get up, binding, size of the book, quality of paper, quality of printing etc., be also taken into consideration.

Importance of Text-books

Text-books occupy a very important place in the teaching of Geography. They form part of the traditional teaching aids. In fact, it would be wrong to call them teaching aids. They are a means of important knowledge. It is through text-books that the knowledge is imparted to students. They serve as a guide and means for the teachers as well as the students. Through the help of the text-books the teacher can impart knowledge to the students and can help them to revise the lesson learnt in the class-room. With the help of the text-books it is also possible to give home-task to the students. If properly used text-books can go a long way in the teaching of Economics in a successful manner.

Utility of Text-books in Primary Classes

In the primary classes the students are not very mature so they require text-books which are capable of serving the under-developed mind. The fact text-book should not be used a lot in primary classes. Text-books be sparingly used in primary classes. Students of primary classes do not require teaching through text-books. They are more interested in listening, the teaching here should be oral. The text-books that are used for the students of these classes should be well-illustrated. They should contain a good number of charts and pictures. They should be written in such a manner that they may serve the psychological requirements of the children of this stage of education.

Text-books in Secondary Classes

Here the students require text-books. Students at this stage of education are properly developed. They are to learn things in a realistic manner. They can benefit a good deal from the text-books. In fact, the method of teaching used at the stage be question-answer method. The students may be asked to read the text-books silently and then questions may be put on the subject-matter. For some difficult subject-matter, the students may be asked to refer to the text-books.

Characteristics and Qualities of Text-books

Text-books in order to be useful should contain the following qualities:

1. Text-books that are intended to be used should be useful for the students as well as the teachers. They should be so designed that on the one hand, they may be written according to the psychological requirements of the students and on the other hand, they should serve the purpose of the teacher who wish to impart knowledge to the students in a successful and interesting manner.
2. The size of the book should be handy. It should be possible for the students to carry them properly. They should not be bulky. This is specially true about books intended for the primary classes.
3. Printing and get up of the books should be interesting and attractive. They should be printed in letters that do not require strain on the eyes of the students. On the other hand, they should be correctly and neatly printed.
4. The exterior of the picture should be attractive. If the exterior is attractive, students should like to carry them and

keep them. This is true of books intended for primary classes.

5. They should serve the purpose of the subject-matter as well as the aims and objects of teaching. They should be written with an eye on the aims and objects of teaching.
6. The text-books should be accurately written. They should present the subject-matter in such a manner that there is no fault in them. The subject-matter, presented therein should be upto date.
7. The style of the book should also serve the psychological requirements of the students of different stages. Text-books intended for the students of primary classes should be written in story form. In the text-books meant for higher classes the author may use a method that is useful for the students at this stage of education.
8. The text-books should continue to keep the interests of the students alive in the subject-matter. The subject-matter should be presented in a simple and lucid style and clear form.
9. The text-books should contain all the necessary and relevant material required for the particular stage of education.
10. The text-books of different stages should be complimentary to each other. Text-books that are used in primary classes should have some bearing and connections with the text-books that shall be used by the students in the junior high school classes.
11. Text-books should be free from prejudice. The presentation of the subject-matter should be unbiased. There should be no material which can injure the susceptibility of any class or category of people. They should contain objective description.
12. At the end of every chapter of the text-book there should be certain questions that may be used for the revision of the subject-matter. Without these questions the text-book shall not be useful.
13. If required the text-books may give a substance of the chapter at the end of each lesson. Such a provision will help the students to grasp the subject-matter properly.

Precautions in regard to Use of Text-books

While the teacher is teaching the students in the class he should not use the text-books very much. Text-books should be used for revising the lesson or for writing out the home-task. The teacher may ask the students to read the book at home or in the class and then put questions in order to ascertain whether the students have grasped the subject-matter or not. While teaching, the teacher must put down substance of the chapter taught on the black-board.

3. Black-board

Black-board is an integral part of the social studies class-room. The black-board should be well-polished and smooth. It should be black in colour and fit for writing with a chalk. In some countries the colour of the black-board has now been made green. This has been done because the green colour is useful for eye-sight. The use of coloured chalk can be made to draw figures, various ways in which black-board is used in teaching of social studies are as follows:

1. It is used for drawing important diagrams.
2. It is used to compare and contrast certain important results. Such results are noted down on black-board.
3. It is used by the teacher to write down certain important points on the black-board to invite the attention of the students to such points.
4. Black-board can also be used for writing down the problems for drill work or assignment etc.
5. Black-board can also be used to plot certain graphs and curves showing various inter-relationships, presenting statistical data etc.

Suggestions for Effective Use of Black-board

For effective use of black-board following points may be given due consideration:

(i) Active cooperation of the students be encouraged to develop the black-board work. If possible the students be encouraged and given opportunity to write and draw on the black-board.

(ii) Coloured chalk may preferably be used.

(iii) The teacher should draw neat diagrams and write legibly on the black-board.

(iv) The teacher should speak while writing on the black-board.

(v) The teacher should take extra precautions not to write anything wrong on the black-board.

(vi) While writing on the black-board teacher should keep an eye on his students.

(vii) The black-board writing should always be in horizontal straight lines.

(viii) Only that portion of the black-board be used for writing which is visible to the students.

4. Flannel-board

Generally the teacher finds it convenient to depict items on the flannel-board. Various items are made out of chart-paper. Pieces of sand paper or cotton are pasted on the back side of each item. Instead of writing with a piece of chalk various items are struck against the surface of the flannel-board.

Flannel-board is useful in depicting certain diagrams, results etc. Particularly when we have to make clear inter-relationsships or continuity of various steps. Flannel-board introduces novelty and change in the class atmosphere.

How to Use a Flannel-board

Following points be kept in mind for effective use of flannel-board:

(i) The teacher should collect a large number of pictures or wall cut diagrams etc., and make use of these one by one after proper selection.

(ii) Display the material on the flannel-board in a sequence to develop the lesson.

(iii) Make proper use of flannel-board in a sequence to develop the lesson.

(iv) Change the material on the board as frequently as possible.

(v) Flannel-board can be used quite effectively for showing relationship between different parts or steps of a process.

Advantages of Flannel-board

Some of the advantages of flannel board are as under :

(i) It is quite economical and easy to handle and operate.

(ii) The pictures or cuttings can be easily fixed and removed when required without spoiling the material. Thus the same material can be used for display many a times.

(iii) Any display material on the board hold the interest of students and arrests their attention.

(iv) Such boards enable a teacher to talk alongwith changing illustrations to develop a lesson.

5. Bulletin-board

It is a display board and has a great value for teaching of social studies. It is used for displaying pictures, drawings, compositions, posters, photographs, newspaper clippings. Such bulletin-boards can be specified for specific branches or topics in social studies. Such a board should be fixed at a conspicuous place in the social studies room. The material displayed should be directly concerned with the activities of the pupils. An effort be made to change the material on bulletin-board as frequently as practicable. Whenever, teacher starts a new topic he may ask the students to display the concerned material on the bulletin-board and the teacher should specifically mention to the students the display material on the board while teaching a topic to the class. Students be asked to take the charge of bulletin-board by rotation.

Social Studies Bulletin-board

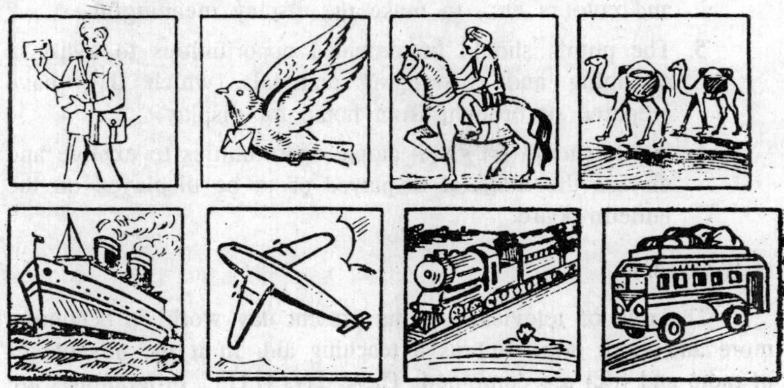

Displays on the bulletin-board should be attractive, appropriate, meaningful, timely and interesting. These may include pictures, posters, pamphlets, cartoons, graphs, maps, charts, diagrams, news items, feature articles, magazine articles, samples of pupils' creative work. Each display should be a unit containing one central theme. Some of this type of displays may be:

1. Life in Indian village,
2. Life in Indian town,
3. Life in Kashmir valley,
4. Tea plantation in India,
5. Jackets of books.

How to Use the Bulletin-board Effectively?

The following guidelines must be carefully noted for the effective use of the bulletin-board:

1. The material to be displayed on the bulletin-board, should be interesting and understandable.
2. The material should, as far as possible, be related to the topics being studied in the class.
3. The material should be changed as purposes and problems change. It should be used to move the unit of study forward in useful directions.
4. Balanced and artistic arrangements should be made with appropriate headings, titles, explanatory notes, mountings and colours etc., to make the display meaningful.
5. The pupils should be provided opportunities to assist in arranging and rearranging materials, which they have prepared or brought from home for display.
6. Pupils should be given ample opportunities to explore and discuss the material displayed or to be displayed on the bulletin-board.

6. Television

The role of television in the present day world is becoming more and more important as a teaching aid. In it the advantages of radio and film are combined. These days U.G.C. programmes are a regular feature on 'Door Darshan'.

It is "medium of mass communication which far surpasses in effectiveness anything our civilization has yet known." It accomplishes certain communicative tasks which are incomparable in their effectiveness.

Television, with its two-fold engagement of the eye and the ear, like the motion pictures, can bring us into contract with events in an exciting and clarifying way. It is a "means by which teachers, parents, children, and all citizens may share a common experience at the same time." It is a versatile vehicle to use a beauty of audio-visual materials.

The potentialities of television in history teaching are enormous. It can transport the places and sites of historical importance which the pupils are unable to visit. It can bring the experts in the classroom not only in voice but in person. It can make available to the classroom rare example of natural or man-made objects.

7. Radio

Television is out of question in poor country like India, but radio can be utilised. Various programmes should be organised for teaching of certain topics of Social Studies through radio. Certain dramas and stories may be broadcast by radio that may give to the students the knowledge of certain topics of Social Studies.

Radio can also serve as an effective aids in teaching of Social Studies. Such lessons may be planned which may be broadcast from the radio and they may provide a background to the knowledge of Social Studies. Special programmes may be designed for students which have a bearing on the subject-matter of social studies. It is also possible to listen to the description of towns and other things on radio. Broadcast talks are now a regular feature of All India Radio.

All India Radio has in its regular feature some programmes meant for school children. In such a programme generally talks on educational matters are broadcast by teacher. Such a talk is quite useful for students as also for social studies teacher. The topic, date and time of broadcast of such are given in advance by All India Radio.

8. Film Projectors and Cinemas

At this stage of education students grow interest in films. This agency may be employed for imparting education of Social Studies to the students. Films depicting various events of Social Study importance, such as elections, may be depicted through films. Working of a democracy may also be shown through films.

Film projectors are the means of showing films. With the help of this instrument a film may be projected right into the class-room.

These are further improvements on the teaching aids discussed so far. These have brought about a revolution in teaching of geography. Geography films are shown to the students to illustrate various topics as also to supplement the class-room teaching. Both type of films have some basic objectives to serve.

Film Strip-projector

It is an improvement on magic lantern and this machine can be used to project many a topics on a single strip. One such strip generally consists of 40-100 separate pictures and such film strips are available on loan from Central Film Library, NCERT, New Delhi. On such a film strip pictures concerning one topic are arranged in a definite order.

This machine can be easily handled by the teacher. The machine is operated by hand and thus can be stopped at the discretion of the teacher whenever, he wants to explain some aspects of a topic being shown on machine.

Micro-projector

This projector is generally operated in a dark room. The projection can be taken on vertical screen whole class is expected to see it. However, such a film cannot be distinctly seen by a student if he is sitting at a distance more than 12 feet from the screen.

Film Projector

This machine is used for showing geography films. Some good

science films on various topics are available and these can be had on loan sometimes even free of charge from the source.

Precautions: The teacher should take the following precautions whenever he wants to use a film projection as a teaching aid:

(i) He should satisfy himself about the lighting management and seating arrangement in the room where such film show is to be given.

(ii) He should himself see the film beforehand.

(iii) He should give a complete background of the film to the students before the actual screening of the film.

(iv) He should see that complete calm and peace is maintained during the screening of the film.

(v) Immediately after the film show, he should invite comments, questions etc., from the students and try to answer all the queries of the students.

(vi) He should encourage some of his students to write articles etc., based on the film show and such articles etc., may be shown on wall magazine, may be printed in school magazine.

9. Tape Recorders and Film Strips

Through tape recorders, speeches of important leaders may be reproduced before the students, may be in the class-room, and through film strips subjects may be made more clear.

10. Diagrams and Graphs

Diagrams represent historical facts and events with the help of visual symbols that convey a number of things within a short space and time. They help to present historical data in an interesting way and captivate attention of the pupils. Many themes such as, sources of history, important battles, administrative systems, comparisons and contrast between religions, life in early civilization may be diagramatically presented.

Graphs are used for representing quantitative data showing comparison, trends, developments and relationships. With the help of simple lines, drawn vertically or horizontally, graphs supply visual imageries for abstract ideas and concepts in history. In the teaching of history the following kinds of graphs may conveniently be used:

(a) *Time Line*: Time line gives linear representation of time. Time is the most abstract concept in history. Time line helps the pupils to gain time sense with the help of space symbols. An event happens at a particular time in history and at a particular place. We are interested to know its exact location on the long and unending line of time. In a time line, the length of time is symbodically represented by a line drawn horizontally or vertically. It gives a visual image of the sequence of events and their relative difference in their occurrence in time. It also helps us in comparing and contrasting and showing mutual relationship between events and happening at different places but at the same time.

The main advantage of time charts and time lines are that they help students to develop a sense of time, to see relationships and to read and study with a purpose. They can focus the attention of the whole class on one audio-visual device. They can be used by graphs or individuals for reporting and review purposes as also for reinforcing learning.

Example of Time Lines

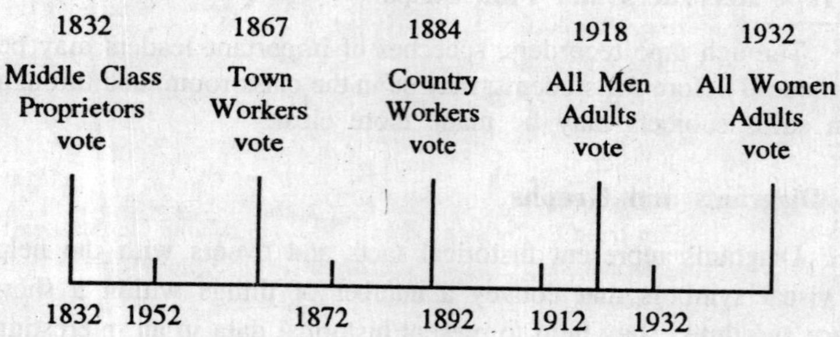

Table Charts

Table Charts: They represent historical data in a tabular form and with their help the pupil gains a comprehensive view of the facts at a sight such charts facilitate comparison and contrast between different historical phenomenon. These charts depend more on language than on symbols.

Examples of Table Charts

Mahatma Gandhi

Decade	Year	Event
1860		
	1869	Birth at Porbunder
1870		
1880		
	1883	Married to Kasturba
	1888	Sent to England
	1891	Called to the Bar
	1892	Went to South Africa
	1899	Served in the Boer War
1900		
	1908	Started Satyagraha in South Africa Imprisoned
1910		
	1912	Gandhi Smuts Pact
	1915	Returned to India Sabarmati Ashram founded
	1919	Rowlatt Act and Jallianwala Bagh Massacre
1920		Started Non-co-operation Movement
	1922	Chauri-Choura Incident
	1924	Elected President of Indian National Congress
1930		Civil Disobedience Movement Dandi March
	1931	Gandhi Irvin Pact Attended Second Round Table Conference
	1932	The Poona Pact
	1935	Sevagram Ashram Founded
1940		
	1942	Quit India Movement
	1944	Kasturba died
	1946	Cabinet Mission
	1947	Indian Independence Act
	1948	Assassinated on 30th January in Delhi
1950		

First-Anglo-Sikh War (1845-46)

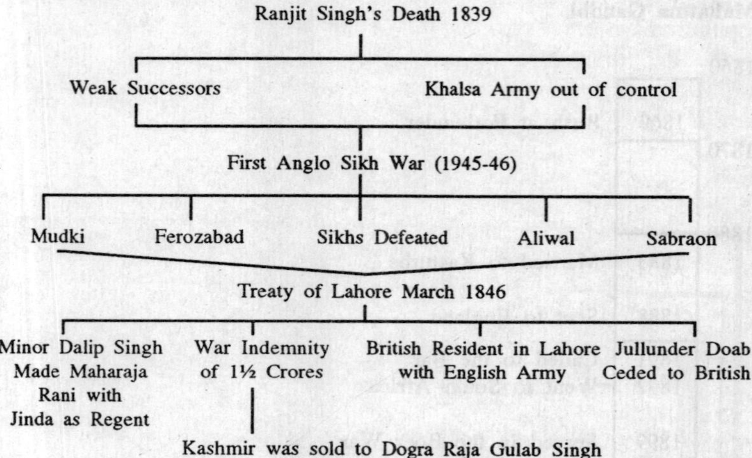

Graphs: Graphs, as used in Social Studies, are a combination of quantitative concepts and factual information of social significance. They are designed to show comparisons, developments, main ideas or relationships clearly so that they can be read and understood quickly. Well-prepared graphs are easy, concise, attractive and limited to most significant facts. The major types of graphs are pictorial, bar, circle and line. Pictorial and bar graphs are easiest to make and to interpret. Circle graphs are best to show relationships of parts to the whole.

Examples of Graphs

1. *Pictorial Graphs:* Showing population of India in comparison to world population.

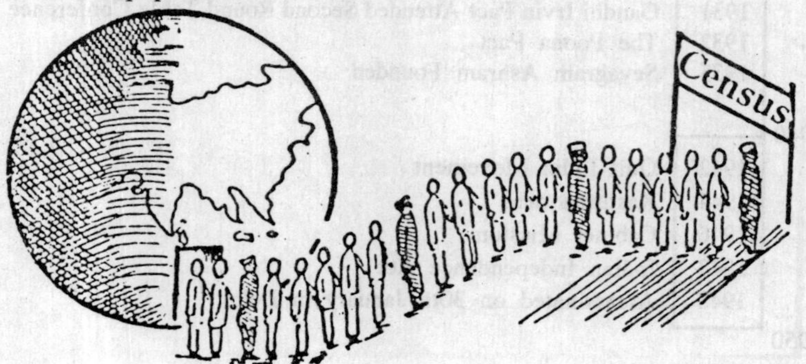

The pictorial graph shows the population of India in relation to world population. India's population is about 1/6th of total world population. So every sixth person in the world is an Indian, as shown in the Pictorial Graph on pre-page.

2. *Bar Graph*

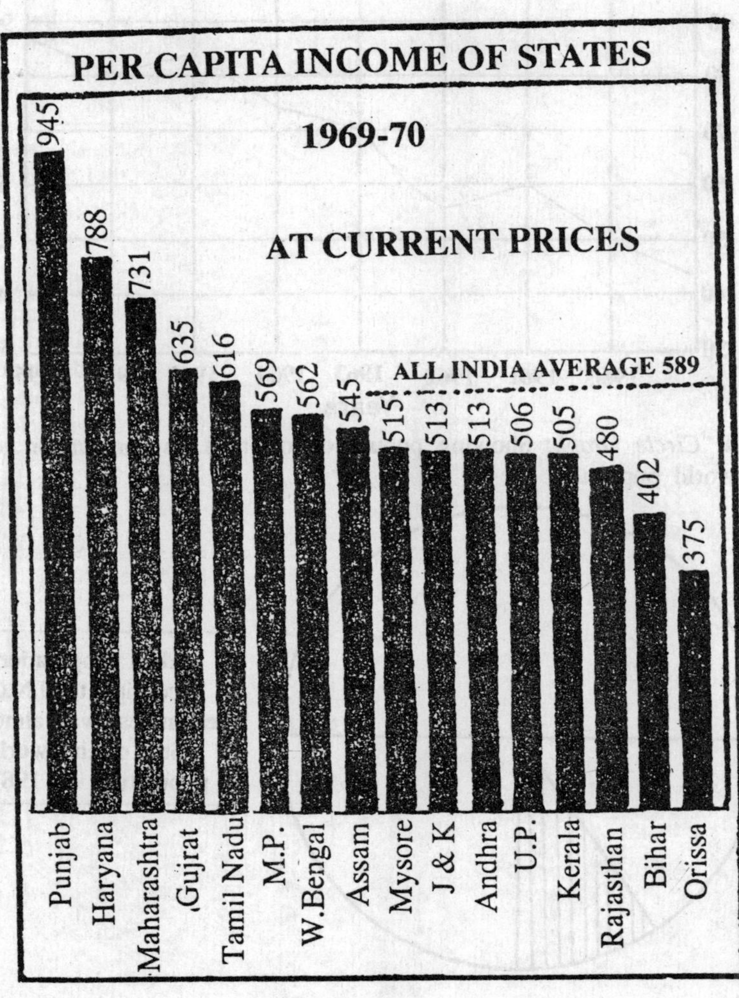

3. *Line Graph:* Showing pass percentage of Matriculation students in a particular school.

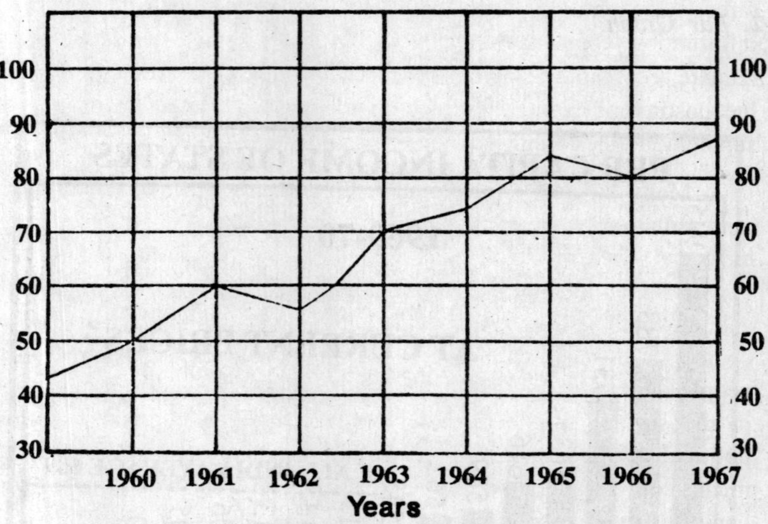

4. *Circle Graph:* Showing population of India, in comparison to world population.

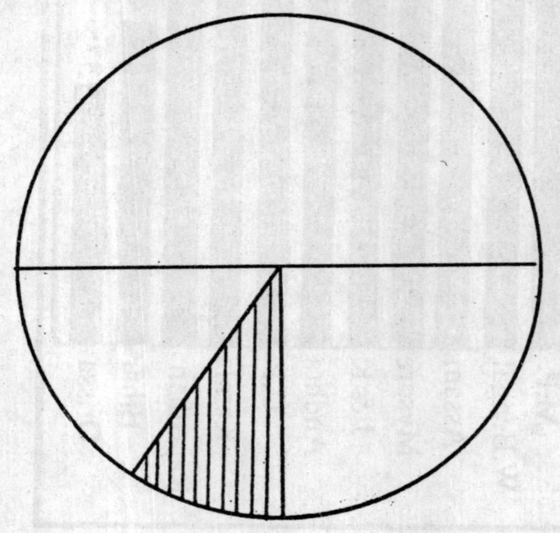

Indian Population according to U.N.O estimates was almost 1/6th of the world population in 1987.

11. Maps

Maps are the universally accepted symbols which represent historical reality in space. They show the location, distance and direction of places connected with historical events. They give information about the distribution of land, water, vegetable life, climate, economic resources which have directly or indirectly shaped the destiny of man. They help to visualise historical realities and supplement their oral and written account.

Maps are of various kinds. Globe gives a three dimensional representation of the earth and may be conveniently used in showing historical events like World Wars I and II and other events of universal character. Relief maps are useful in showing the depressions and elevations on the surface of earth which have influenced the course of history. Invasions, military operations, migration of the people and social intercourse, all bear the impact of the inequalities in the surface of the earth. Flat maps showing physical features, political divisions, population, rainfall, temperature, soil, vegetation, means of transport and communication of the world and other countries provide ample opportunities for illustrating a history lesson.

The teacher tries to substantiate his statements and narration with the help of these maps. He tries to explain various places of historical importance with the help of these maps. Empires of various rulers may be indicated with the help of these maps.

The teacher has to use a pointed for indicating things on the maps. The pointer should be quite pointed at the end so that there may not be any confusion with regard to the location of the place, that the teacher wishes to point out.

The maps should be so drawn and coloured that they may be clearly visible to the students. Writing about maps a scholar says, "The map is not merely an aid to history teaching. It is as essential as in the fundamentals in other works are to be understood. Only through the use of maps can the area and relative positions of political units be visualized and make it possible to indicate the development of states. The progress of military campaigns or of exploration or the general distinction of religions and languages."

Some Important Map Symbols

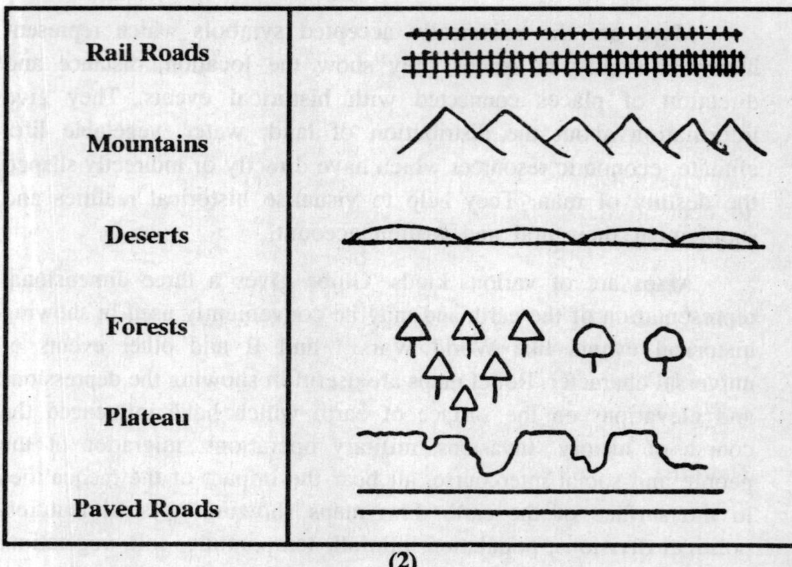

(2)

Rainfall Per Year Shown on the Map	
	Less than 5 inches
	5 to 10 inches
	10 to 20 inches
	20 to 50 inches
	More than 50 inches

12. Models

Since original materials are scarce and rare and even those that exist are beyond the reach of all schools, the history teacher may take the help of models to give as vivid a picture of historical objects as possible. *Model* is nothing but a replica of a thing that we want to present or explain. It makes the teaching of history interesting and gives concrete idea of the abstract things. Models can be used to depict different aspects of human life -- political, economic, social, religious and cultural.

Making of models provides an opportunity for 'learning by doing' and enlivens the interest of the pupils in the topic. Models prepared by the students or purchased from the market should be properly labelled, mounted and displayed. Labels should be short and self-explanatory.

Qualities of a Model

(i) It should be simple to understand.

(ii) It should be useful.

(iii) It should be accurately drawn.

13. Globe

The globe is the most accurate representation of the earth which is available in the class-room. It is a simple but inexhaustible source of help to the students. It is, in fact, a combination of a model and a map. It is really a map with a curved surface and is, therefore, a more accurate reproduction than the one with a flat surface. The globe simplifies the mysteries of the world. No device can be more helpful in expanding one's conception of the earth than the globe. It gives us the correct concept of the Arctic and Antarctic circles, the Axis of the earth, hemispheres, latitudes, longitudes, meridian, prime-meridian and the poles. The phenomena of seasons and rotations and revolutions of the earth can be explained with the help of a globe. Similarly, location and relationship of different parts of the world and land and sea routes etc. can be taught and understood clearly through the globe.

Maps used in conjunction with the globe are very valuable instructional material in Social Studies. But pupils should be taught to get correct information from the globe and the maps. They should be able to locate countries, mountains and rivers etc. For understanding modern complex society the comparison and contrast of different areas of the world is very important. But that is possible only if pupils have been taught how to read and interpret the globe and the maps and when they have got adequate understanding of them.

The globe should be used to develop fundamental concepts about the earth and its surface features. In primary classes, the globe may be used to develop concepts of the roundness of the earth, directions, how three-fourths of earth's surface is covered by water, how surface features differ from place to place and how major land areas and water bodies differ in size. In secondary classes the globe may be used to develop concepts of the formation of day and night, changes in seasons, rotation and revolution of the earth and latitudes and longitudes. Concept development of this kind is essential to the development of map-reading and map drawing skills, so useful for understanding major geographic concepts.

14. Histrionics

Histrionics include dramas, plays, pageants, tableaux, mock-performances and soliloquies etc. Indian history and literature are full of ready-made histrionics which can throw a flood of light on various phases in Social Studies. Such activities provide scope for expression and imagination. They sharpen learning, appeal to emotions and to a great extent, help in removing inferiority complex. They provide rich experiences to children to show their resourcefulness, enthusiasm and excitement for action. They create interest and exercise initiative and originality of children and leave deep impression on young minds. They not only teach proper intonation and pronunciation, but also provide opportunities for planning, organising and executing a project. At the junior high school stage pupils should be encouraged to write dialogues, prepare costumes and scenery and to investigate thoroughly the events to be dramatised. It should, however, be noted that dramatisation should be simple and its instructional value should be paramount throughout. At the higher secondary stage level, the materials may be represented as a radioscript or it may asssume the shape of a mock performance, a debate or a penal discussion.

15. Social Studies Laboratory

Children are eager collectors. They can help a lot in collecting various articles of use and interest which can be kept and exhibited in the laboratory. No doubt a lot of knowledge can be had from arranging educational trips to museums owned by various State Governments. But each secondary school should try to build its own Social Studies laboratory to meet the new demands of modern education. But pupils and teachers can collect a large number of articles, suitable for the laboratory and this should be considered a definite part of the educational programme. In a laboratory we can have models of various projects, going on in the country, models of castles, temples, monasteries, palaces and old buildings; charts showing evolution of various aspects of national life, pictures, maps drawings, graphs, diagrams, stamps, coins, tools, implements and several other things which can be collected with the help of students. Old letters, pictures, news-papers, journals, records, manuscripts, statues, coins and such other things which can be collected without much difficulty. A well-organised laboratory which contains objects to illustrate different periods of the past, often results in greatly increased interest in Social Studies. All objects, specimens, and models should be carefully classified and labelled. Whenever, the exhibition of an article is desired for a class, it must be accompanied by discussion or explanation. This will lead to better understanding and a greater appreciation of the topic in hand. But all the exhibits in the laboratory should be easily moveable and easily available for instructional purposes, whenever needed.

16. Resource Visitors

For the effective teaching of Social Studies, it is educationally very sound if different job-men like the Chairman of the local Municipal Committee, the Sarpanch of the Local Panchayat, local Police Inspector, the Bank Manager, the Post-Master, the Station Master, the M.L.A. of the area and other such persons are invited to the school. They can explain effectively the importance of their own jobs and how they are of help to society in their own sphere. They would, thus, extend the knowledge of school children, about the multiple activities of society. The children will learn how people, engaged in different jobs and vocations, are contributing to the welfare of the society. They will realise that a sweeper, a porter or a stone-breaker is as useful to society as a doctor, a teacher or a magistrate.

17. Celebration of Festivals, Fairs and National Days

Utilization of fairs, festivals and national days, celebrated in India, can serve as a very important device of teaching Social Studies. Whenever birth or death anniversaries of great Indian heroes and heroines are celebrated or whenever a religious, seasonal or national festival comes, the children are very eager to know its significance. On such occasions it is the duty of the teacher to throw light on the lives of those great personalities and also to explain the importance of various festivals in the life of our nation. This will enable the students to realize how great men and women of their country have contributed to the welfare and uplift of their countrymen and what their own duty is towards the community. This will also help in developing among children the noble attitudes of toleration, fellow-feeling, co-operation and self-sacrifice. Similarly, birth-days of great teachers and leaders of other countries who have contributed to world movements and universal peace, should also be celebrated in the school. National days like the Independence Day, the Republic and the Teachers' Day and international days like the United Nations Day and the Human Rights Day should also be celebrated with great advantage, in the school.

Audio-Visual Aids and the Social Studies Teacher

The great importance of audio-visual material as aids to teaching cannot be doubted. But a word of caution is necessary in regard to their use. Some people think that the importance of these new aids to teaching is increasing so rapidly that a day may come when these will take the place of the teacher. This is absolutely wrong. Teaching is strictly a personal affair between the teacher and the pupil. It is a contact of mind and mind. As such, no apparatus, device or aid can replace the teacher. In fact, there is no such thing as **audio-visual education**. There are only **audio-visual aids of education**. As such, the new devices, however, extensive their appeal and intensive their motivation may be, must be regarded as **aids to learning.** Their primary purpose is to provide variety in the techniques of teaching and thus vitalise the procedure. They are merely supplementary devices at the disposal of the teacher, to be used as and when he deems proper. Their sole aim is to widen the already existing interest of the pupils. There is yet another wrong impression that audio-visual aids are the luxury of the imperialist government and that they are an attempt to hide bad teaching. Such fears are unfounded and baseless. These aids are not the fads of the modernists, nor they are meant for hiding bad teaching. They are something usual and natural and should be employed in full context to one point or points in the lesson in order to vitalize the teaching-learning process.

It is also equally wrong to pressume that the job of the motion picture or a slide, or a film-strip or a broadcast is over as soon as it has been displayed or listened to. The work of the teacher, in fact, begins where the picture ends or the broadcast finishes. This is because these aids have to be used as means to further activity instead of regarding them as ends in themselves. Moreover, they should not be used for developing passive receptivity in the pupils by virtue of their being interesting and entertaining. They have to be used only as devices for stimulating learning. It is also important to note that there should be no over-emphasis on their use. They should not be used for the sake of using them but only when they are actually needed and when they are relevant to the topic and suitable to the age and experience of the pupils.

It should also be remembered by teachers that just as there is no one way of bringing up babies, similarly, there is no one way of using these devices for teaching purposes. Teaching is not mere telling or displaying of certain material. It is a personal affair between the teacher and the pupil. It is, therefore, absolutely essential that any system of teaching must be elastic enough to give freedom in modifying techniques. There are hundreds and thousands of such techniques, most of which are the result of the teacher's own thinking, initiative and resourcefulness. A teacher may be an adept in one device and a failure in another. But whatever devices he uses, these should give variety, create interest, stimulate thinking, provide outlets for hidden talent and reveal the temperaments of students. These must help the pupils in motivating their learning and developing new interests in them. The teacher must plan ways and means to encourage pupil's expression of reactions in order to realise a more valuable experience from the audio-visual materials.

Teachers of Social Studies should also note that aids must be appropriate for the age, intelligence and experience of the learners. Audio-visual aids may be profusely used in lower classes. But as pupils grow, they develop imagination and therefore, the need for such devices in higher classes decreases.

6.8 MAIN ADVANTAGES OF THE AUDIO-VISUAL AIDS

(i) Best motivators.
(ii) Fundamental to verbal instructions.
(iii) Clear images.
(iv) Vicarious experience.
(v) Variety.
(vi) Freedom.
(vii) Opportunity to handle and manipulate.

6.9 PROBLEMS IN THE USE OF TEACHING AIDS

Though these aids are becoming more and more popular every day yet there are certain problems that are faced and must be solved. These are:

(i) Apathy of the Teachers

Teachers are not yet convinced that teaching with words alone is quite tedious, wasteful and ineffective.

(ii) Indifference of Students

The judicious use of aids arouses interest but if used without a definite purpose they lose their significance and importance.

(iii) Ineffectiveness of the Aids

Because of the absence of proper planning and the lethargy of the teacher and without proper preparation, correct presentation, appropriate application and discussion and the essential follow up work, the aids have not proved their full usefulness. A film like a good lesson has various steps--preparation, presentation, application and discussion.

(iv) Financial Hurdles

The central and state governments have set up Boards of Audio-visual Education and have chalked out interesting programmes for the popularisation of teaching aids but the lack of finances has not enabled them to do their best.

(v) Absence of Electricity

Most of the projectors cannot work in the absence of electricity which is not readily available these days.

(vi) Lack of Facilities for Training

At present we do not have sufficient number of training institutes and more and more teaching colleges or specialised agencies should be opened to train teachers and workers in the use and usefulness of these aids.

(vii) Co-ordination between Centre and States

Good film libraries, museums of audio-visual education, fixed and mobile exhibitions and educational 'melas' should be organised both by centre and the states.

(vii) Language Difficulty

Most films are in English. We should have them in Hindi and other Indian languages.

(ix) Not Catering to Local Needs

No attention is paid in the production of Audio-visual aids to the sociological, psychological and pedagogical factors.

(x) Improper Selection of Films

Films are not selected according to the Class-room needs.

6.10 FUTURE OF TEACHING AIDS

Today, the problem is not whether visual aids should have a place in education. This has been recognised long ago. The problem, now, is that of extending the benefits of the teaching aids to all the teachers and students. The future of these aids can be bright if we make a proper planning and carry out good co-ordination between producers, teachers and students. Useful and effective aids can be produced only after getting the reaction of the audience and by carrying out a good deal of research work in the field.

REVIEW QUESTIONS

1. What kinds of material aids would you suggest in the teaching of Social Studies to inculcate civic ideals among the students and why?
2. To what extent should radio and tape recording be based in teaching social studies?
3. How can teaching aids be justified in teaching of social studies?
4. Discuss the use of maps in social studies.
5. Discuss the different aids that a social studies teacher should employ to make his subject interesting.
6. Define audio-visual aids and give main reasons for their use.
7. Discuss the importance of following in the teaching of social studies.

   (i) Charts,

   (ii) Motion pictures,

   (iii) Diagrams, and

   (iv) Pictures.

7

Utilizing Current Affairs

7.1 INTRODUCTION

At present current affairs is included as a part of curriculum in schools. "Current affairs" includes "current events" and "current issues" or problems.

"Current events" are historical and deal with already settled problems whereas "current issues" are the problems which are now under consideration and they may or may not be solved in near future.

In social studies current affairs are more significant as they represent "an extension and an exemplification of the major topics in curriculum". In the words of R.S. Kimbal, current affairs, "is a field which is concerned with all those happenings, both domestic and international, social, political or economic, a knowledge and understanding of which is necessary as a basis for a citizenship of loyalty and service."

Current affairs should not form a separate topic but it be taught as an integral part of study of each unit.

7.2 IMPORTANCE OF CURRENT AFFAIRS

One of the important aims of education, these days, is to produce democratic citizens and the training in the habits for citizenship, can best be achieved through the study of current affairs. The study of current affairs is quite helpful to the pupil to learn how to discuss and evaluate world happenings in the light of past history and present situations. It also make it clear that the present age is age of internationalism. In the present age every one of us must be fully aware of the latest happening not only within his country but the world over. One should show sympathy, tolerance, fellow feeling, cooperation, selflessness and mutual understanding all the times. The study of current affairs also enables the pupil to understand changes in future society and to adjust himself in accordance with such changes. A study in current affairs equips the individual to face problems boldly and to think of their solutions intelligently. It also helps him to learn how to select, defend, present and modify his own point of view. We thus conclude that the study of current affairs is important for training in dynamic citizenship.

7.3 PURPOSE OF TEACHING CURRENT AFFAIRS

The inclusion of current affairs in school curriculum serves the following purposes:

1. It promotes interest in current affairs and news development. It helps to keep the individual upto date on the rapidly changing course of events. Its study helps to promote interest in world happenings.
2. It promotes the growth of certain desirable skills and abilities such as:
   (i) the ability and skill of reading the news material;
   (ii) the ability to distinguish between more important and less important news-items;
   (iii) the ability to take a position on conflicting issues; and
   (iv) the ability to foretell the likely consequences in terms of present developments.

   The development of such fundamental skills and abilities is a must if any individual has to exercise critical judgement about current affairs.
3. A course in current affairs is helpful to the child in relating school learnings to life outside the school. The revision of text-books and reference books takes sometime and a study of current affairs is thus quite essential to make social studies upto date and more functional.

O. Columbus, in his pamphlet on "Discussion and Current Affairs", has given the following main purposes of current affairs instruction in schools:

1. To help pupils to identify important problems and issues to see how these affect their lives and to sense what they can do about them.
2. To help pupils recognise and respect democratic values in reacting to processes, problems and issues.
3. To encourage pupils to develop habits of and a continued interest in reading, listening, enquiring and observing as ways of keeping informed about current affairs.
4. To help pupils acquire the greatest possible proficiency in the skills, needed for obtaining and using social information.
5. To help pupils acquire proficiency in locating, organising and evaluating information on important issues and in evaluating and analysing the judgement of others on these issues.
6. To encourage pupils to "put themselves in the shoes" of other people in evaluating their way of life and their position in problems and issues.
7. To help pupils to develop facility in the democratic discussion of issues, orally and in writing.
8. To help pupils to see the importance of revising judgements in the light of new evidence.
9. To afford pupils a variety of opportunities for action to implement conclusions, reached on important issues.

7.4 CRITERIA FOR SELECTING CURRENT EVENTS

1. Suitability

While selecting news-items for pupils, their age, experience and understanding should be kept in view. Only such items be selected which are quite suitable for the standard of the class and which can really add to the knowledge of the child.

2. Reliability

The events included should be quite reliable and accurate.

3. Scope

Only the items with wide scope be included in curriculum. However, sometime a local event may become international in scope.

The teacher is expected to evaluate the importance of an item in terms of scope before selecting it.

4. Recency

It is this quality that differentiates "current affairs" from the rest of the curriculum. This applies to latest discoveries, inventions etc. A knowledge of these helps an individual to understand the social changes that these are likely to produce.

5. Utility

Only such news items be selected which are of some utility to the students, e.g. weather forecast, business reports, sports news etc.

6. Notability

In selection of news items the teacher should always keep in mind that the news concerning some big countries or concerning some important personalities are more significant and so due consideration has to be given to this fact.

7. Consequence

It refers to the effect of some news on report in the press. A news may be considered quite important if it reports some sudden or radical change. In its consequence a report-calling for some immediate action may be considered more important than others.

8. Continuity

Those news which show the continuing process of social adjustment in modern life may be given preference. In this category we may include news items relating to, the art of government, achieving national independence, securing religious rights, election campaign, session of political parties, strikes, labour laws etc.

However, these are only guidelines and actually there are no hard and fast rules for the selection of news items for school children. The only criterion is that these should be suitable and reliable. In selecting them more than one criterion be used instead of any one criterion.

7.5 PROGRAMME OF CURRENT AFFAIRS INSTRUCTIONS

As has already been made clear there is no need to include such a programme separately in the curriculum and that it should be taught as an integral part of the different units in social studies classes.

Here we suggest a few ways of including current affairs in the school programme.

1. Teaching Current Affairs in Addition to Social Studies

In most of our schools we have morning assembly in which the staff and students are required to be present. Just after prayers etc., it would be appropriate to spare a few minutes for discussion on important news-items or announcement of important news items. The cuttings of such news may also be displayed on the bulletin-board.

2. To Use the Current Affairs for Supplementing the Teaching of Social Studies

While discussing any specific unit in social studies the teacher should cite the news items related to that topic. Even students be encouraged to look out for any related news and to use the same to make their knowledge upto date. Such material may also be put up on the bulletin-board. It may be a news article, magazine article, etc.

3. Using Current Affairs as a Basis of Social Studies Unit

It is an ideal if any unit on Social Studies can be developed around some current affair. However utmost care must be taken to select such a unit because it is quite possible that the books may not contain much of the material dealing with the topic in the news. This can be tried for units dealing with progress in science, technology, medicine, industry, education etc. Current affairs as starting point for these is likely to stimulate more interest among the students.

To get the best results it is better to make use of all the three procedures outlined above and the teacher may follow them as the occasion demands.

7.6 USE OF VARIOUS LEARNING ACTIVITIES IN CURRENT AFFAIRS PROGRAMME

It is possible to make use of various learning activities in the current affairs programme. Some of the activities that can be profitably used are as follows:

1. Panel Discussion

The total number of participants in such a discussion is 4-8 persons including a chairman. The person participating in it represent large group and the aim is to provide the features of a small group for the benefit of a large group.

Such a discussion may be held on stage or on raised plateform on which the seats for participants may be arranged in a semi-circular form to facilitate them being heard and seen by the audience. Chairman opens such a discussion. He explains the whole problem and coordinates the discussion and brings to a close the panel discussion by summarising the proceedings. In such a discussion listners are also given an opportunity to ask questions and make contributions. In such a discussion long speeches and debates are not allowed.

At the end of the discussion, the chairman of the panel summarises the entire topic in an integrated form.

2. Round Table Discussion

It is an open type of discussion in which the whole class participates. Sometimes the class may be divided into 4-5 discussion groups so as to clarify the same topic. It is felt that a discussion in smaller groups is more effective. After discussion each group presents a short summary of the important points and this is put before the whole class.

3. Preparation of Maps, Charts and Graphs

The pupils may be asked to prepare maps, charts or graphs to illustrate various current events. Outline maps be used and important news and events may be inserted at their proper places. Graphs showing rise and fall in population, employment, production, export, import etc. may be exhibited. Charts or even posters may be prepared showing progress in space travels, changes in air travel etc.

4. Keeping Newspaper Cuttings, Cartoons and Pictures in Scrap-books

Teacher may encourage his students to collect important cartoons, pictures and head-line cuttings related to units in social studies and keep them in their scrap-books, note-books for study and reference. It is quite a useful activity.

5. Reporting News

Teacher may assign to the selected students the duties to collect weekly news related to certain topics. These news may then be reported to the whole class in the weekly meetings. By this activity the child gets a training in selecting, planning and presenting reports before a gathering of educated persons.

6. Dramatising News-items

Some of the news particularly those that deal with festivals, conferences, meetings etc., can be dramatised. It will add to the pupils interest in the current affairs.

7.7. SPECIMEN CURRENT AFFAIRS FOR HIGH CLASSES

Following are some of the current affairs which would be beneficial for students of High classes.

1. General Elections

In any democratic country the government of the country is formed through general elections and this activity is a good and effective means of teaching to the students the formation of central and state governments. It can also be used to show the working of governments in a welfare society.

2. Election of the President

In most of the democracies the President is the head of the state and how he is elected will be an interesting activity for high class students. With the help of this activity the students may be taught the duties and rights of the President in a democratic country. In this activity the teacher can also discuss the policies of the newly formed governments.

3. Interplanetary Space Travels

Man has landed on moon and has planned travels to Mars and other planets. All this has been possible due to progress in science and technology. With the help of this activity the teacher can bring home, to the students, various advances in science and technology and their use for the mankind.

4. Discord between Two Countries

Though the UNO has been trying its best to maintain peace and harmony in the world yet we find that a number of discords exist and sometimes it leads to a military action by one country against the other for settlement of some pending dispute. Taking any such current affair teacher can easily explain that the use of force is not advisable to solve any national or international problem. It is always desirable to solve all pending disputes by mutual understanding and self-restraint.

5. International Conferences and Meetings

In News are always such international conferences and meeting where the current affairs are discussed. Teacher can make use of such a news item to explain to his students, how representatives of various nations meet and discuss various problems. He should concentrate his efforts to bring to the notice of his students, the praise worthy efforts made by UNESCO, ILO, WHO, IMF etc.

6. Some Interesting Judicial Case

We always find certain interesting news items concerned with the legal system of the country, making use of such news items the teacher can tell his students the difference between the civil case and the criminal case, the functions of various courts such as Lower Courts, District Courts, High Courts and the Supreme Court. Students be made to understand clearly the distinction between judiciary, legislature and executive. If possible and appropriate the functions of International Court of Justice may also be explained.

7. Visit of a Foreign Dignitary

In this age of internationalism the visit of foreign dignitaries is quite frequent and the news of such a visit can be used by the social studies teacher to explain such topics that deal with international peace and understanding, good relations between nation etc.

8. Celebration of National and International Day

The celebration of national and international day is an appropriate occasion to study the life and contribution of a national hero. Such an occasion can also be used by the Social Studies teacher to give information concerning India's struggle for Independence and its achievements thereafter. Teacher can explain the function of UNO and its various agencies while celebrating some international day.

7.8. THE ROLE OF THE TEACHER

The programme in current affairs is to be formulated by the Social Studies teacher and so he is the key figure. His role as a guide and leader is indispensable. To perform this role efficiently and effectively the foremost requirement is that the social studies teacher is well-informed about the current affairs, contemporary problems and their possible solutions. The observations by R. S. Kimbal in this respect are important. He observes, "Current events can be taught successfully when a teacher is sufficiently interested himself. The varying degrees of success however seem to indicate that the ability of the teacher, rather than the quality of the medium or the method, is the determining factor. Almost any device can be used effectively. The teacher's own interest, his own enthusiasm, his own understanding of what should be accomplished, are the matters which determine the failure or success of current events teaching. The best available media fail in their purpose when used by class guided by a teacher unskilled in methods of current events instructions. The poorest seem to accord some measure of success when a capable current event teacher works with his pupils."

REVISION QUESTIONS

1. Mention different ways in which the current affairs be included in school programme.
2. Discuss the importance of Newspapers as a teaching aid in Social Studies.
3. Give an outline of the various criterion to be used for selecting "current affairs" for various school classes.
4. Discuss some activities which, in your opinion, may prove useful for studying "current affairs."
5. What are "current affairs?" Discuss their importance in teaching of Social Studies.

8

Utilizing Community Resources

8.1 INTRODUCTION

A new trend that is visible in our educational programme, these days, is the central role assigned to the community. It is now emphasised that the education should be of the community, by the community and for the community. This aim can be achieved by bringing the community and school closer to each other. If we want to make education, a living experience for the children then it is possible only if the education is given in community at large instead of our schools. Most of his time is spent by the child in community and so it is desirable to make the community as a laboratory for the child, where an effort be made to give the child a large number of living experiences.

This reorientation will provide the nation the vigour, life and power, which will help to sustain not any individual but also the nation as a whole. To bring about this reorientation the schools have to give up their isolation and adopt a new role i.e., the role of community schools. It requires that the barrier between school and community be broken and a bridge to constructed for continuous flow of traffic between the school and the community. Such a flow will help each other and the school and community will be complementary to each other. For achieving a unification between the school and the community we may allow the *direct participation of school in community life*. With such a participation school may help to provide solution to vital problems, confronting the community.

In the words of K.G. Saiyidain, "A Community school must obviously be based on the community needs and problems. Its curriculum should be an epitome of community life. It should reflect all that is significant and characteristic in life of the community in its natural setting."

8.2 COMMUNITY AS AN IMPORTANT SOURCE OF EDUCATION

Community is the most important resource for the education of the child. It is the child's laboratory. It provides the child the first hand learning experiences about the ways of living. It is through his active participation in community life that a child learns and develops the basic concepts of history, geography, economics, transportation, communication etc., including various aspects of living in a community. The community life provides the child various opportunities which help the child develop an insight into the reasons and conditions which contribute to changes in social life. From such experiences child makes generalisations about his community and tries to make a comparison between the ways of living of his community with those of some other communities. A larger number of experiences of the child with his own community helps him to understand in a better way the ways of living in other places and other communities which may be living in different parts of the world.

The community is a treasure house of rich and varied source and can so it can enrich and supplement learning in Social Studies. To fully utilize the community resources an important role has to be played by teachers, administrators, local citizens, parents and pupils. Only a well-planned programme can bring both the school and community close to each other. The programme be planned in such a way that it brings the school and community quite close to each other. The first hand knowledge that a child acquires by his community experiences helps him in becoming an intelligent citizen.

The community provides a connection between the past and the present and it inspires men everywhere. It has a dignity and a meaning. If teacher fails to make full use of the community in which his school is situated than he is over-looking one of the richest sources of education for his pupils.

For utilizing the community resources fully the school should take itself to the community and consider the community as a big laboratory for the education of its pupils. An all out effort be made to discover the community resources, understand its culture, appreciate its problems and to provide solutions to the problems of the community. While working in community the student gets opportunity to explore not only physical setting but also the human setting.

In physical setting are included size, climate, topography, soil, numerals and other similar problems. In human setting are included the people inhabitating that community. It will also include those problems that relate to population, health, education, occupation and other considerations that-result in class and caste structures. For carrying out such studies it is essential to carry out a thorough survey of the community and complete utilization of its resources for educative purposes.

8.3 THE NEED FOR SCHOOL-COMMUNITY RELATIONSHIP

The School is the product of community which is called upon to serve. It has been rightly said that, ''Community builds its schools and schools build their community. In this connection, Prof. Ryburn has opined.

"There must be a vital connection between the life of the pupils in school and the life of the community from which they come. Their must be a vital connection between the school which is the corporate life of pupils, teachers and community, otherwise the school can never succeed in its aim of enabling its pupils to get out and to face society and make necessary adjustment nor can it, as a corporate body, even have the vital influence on the community which it ought to have.''

This observation clearly brings about the interdependence of school and community in each other. Thus it is essential for the two to work in close adjustment with each other.

Stressing the need for school-community relationship, the Secondary Education Commission has remarked, ''we should in the first place, take due note of the fact that the school is a small community, within a larger community and that the attitudes, values and modes of behaviour—good or bad—which have currency in national life are bound to be reflected in school.''

In the words of K.G. Saiyiadin ''School Community Cooperation is really something more basic than parent, teacher or student community relationship ... if there is no living, dynamic relationship between the two, education will be enormic, unreal, unable to make an abiding impact on the mind and character of the children.''

Thus unless right points of contact are established between school and community, education would remain ineffective and artificial, incapable of being utilized as an instrument of social progress.

For strengthening the relationship between the school and the community following suggestions be given due consideration:

1. Decentralise education and the right persons from community be allowed due participation in the management of schools.
2. Each school should have a local advisory committee consisting of notable persons of the community. Their function is only to advise and not to interfere.
3. Important and respectable members from community be extended invitations to attend important school functions.
4. "Parent Day" be organised every year in the school.
5. "Parent-Teacher Assiociation" can be one of the vital instruments that can help in strengthening the relationship between the school and the community.
6. School building be placed at the disposal of the community on important social occasions.
7. Arrangements be made to start adult education classes in schools in the evening hours.
8. Allow the use of school library to members of the community during evening hours.
9. Now and then the school should organise a film show, drama, nutrition show, child care show etc., for the benefit of the community.
10. It is also possible to organise community games in the schools.
11. Schools can run a vocational guidance centre for the members of the community.

These can be summed up in the words of Secondary Education Commission, "What we should like to see in a two way traffic so that the problems that arise in the home and community life and the realistic experiences gained should be brought into school so that education may be based on them and be intimately connected with real life and on the other hand, the new knowledge, skills, attitudes and values acquired in the school should be carried into the home life to solve its problems, to raise its standards and link up the teachers, parents and children in one compact and naturally helpful group."

8.4 IMPORTANT COMMUNITY RESOURCES

To make best use of the available community resources, the teacher should help his pupils to catalogue the available resources before proceeding to study them. The catalogue should include every information available about the places that can enrich instructions in Social Studies. Each place be listed separately with maximum possible information about its name, location, route to reach the place, persons to be contacted, most appropriate time to visit the place, the resources and materials of study available, expenses likely to be incurred etc.

For preparing the catalogue readily usable it may be divided into various sections as follows:

1. Places of Historical Interest

This section may include various temples, churches, Gurdwaras, mosques, old historical records, building, monuments etc.

2. Places of Geographical Interest

It may include such places as factories, mills, railway station, sea-ports, air-ports, telephone exchange, radio station, TV centre, theatres etc.

3. Places of Social and Cultural Interest

This list may include various clubs, parks, museums, zoo, art galleries, fun and food resorts, university etc.

4. Places of Economic Interest

It includes banks, trading centres, stock exchange, markets, kilns, dairies, LIC buildings etc.

5. Government Buildings

In this section should be included the Panchayat Ghar, Hospital,

Police Station, Water Supply, Community Centre, various government offices etc.

6. A separate section be spared to catalogue traditions, customs, rituals, ceremonies, practices, beliefs, attitudes etc., of the local community.

8.5 UTILIZATION OF COMMUNITY RESOURCES

The available community resources be utilized for bringing the community to the school and by taking the school to the community.

1. Taking the School to the Community

If students are given an opportunity to observe the environment where they live, it will help them to view history in its proper perspective and the geography as it exists. Such an opportunity will be utilized by them to know about people and their occupations and business and industries that comprise that community. They get first hand information of different activities of the community. Such an opportunity can be provided to the students in any of the following ways:

(a) Field Trips and Excursions

The organisation of field trips and excursions has been discussed at length in another chapter. It would suffice here to add that students are always ready for such trips. Such a trip will help in understanding of the topic or the problem by direct observation. Such a field trip may be useful to the students as it may enable them to recognise flowers, plants, trees, birds, cattles etc. which they may come across during their trip. They will also be able to observe various irrigation facilities, roads, means of transport, agricultural crops, various industrial units, trade centre, places of economic interest etc. during such a visit. It will help them to know much more about the life of the community.

(b) Community Survey

Community surveys of a particular nature may be undertaken by the senior students of the school. Such a survey may be conducted to study the past history of the community, present position of the community, economic condition of the community, etc. Survey can also be conducted about the social institutions, traditions, customs, ceremonies, folk lores, folk dances, habits etc., prevalent in the community.

Even the common problems such as housing, unemployment, poverty, child labour, place of women etc. can form the topic of a survey.

For conducting survey the students can take help from social workers, elders of the society, government officials etc. They can consult maps, charts, records, documents available and may visit certain places, buildings, offices, factories etc., to get more information. These surveys will be quite helpful to chart a future course of action.

(c) Organisation of Relief Services

School students may take a lead in organising relief services in the community. However all such services be organised only under the guidance and supervision of a teacher. Such relief services can be organised at the times of natural calamities such as floods, earth quake, epidemic etc.

(d) Organising Health-squads and Social Service

Students can render service to the community by extending their help in the form of volunteers on such occasions as fairs, festivals, elections etc. They can also help the community by undertaking social service programmes such as cleaning the lanes, streets, drains, drinking water wells, surroundings etc. They can also undertake to beautify the surroundings, tree plantation, etc.

They can even help the needy persons in hospitals, post-office, banks etc. They can definitely undertake adult education programme and contribute in the literacy programme of the country.

2. Bringing the Community to the School

This can be done in the following ways:

(a) Parent Teacher Association

Parent Teacher Association plays an important role in strengthening the relationship between the school and the community. In order to have a permanent exchange of views between the school and the home-- the two vital agencies of education-- Parent-teacher association should become a vital instrument in bringing community and the school closer to each other.

Parent-teacher association should meet at regular intervals and discuss the important educational problems relating to the child, the school and the home. It is a sad fact that such associations are given little importance in Indian schools while most of the traditional schools prefer in isolation from the community. But the real need is that each and every school pupil should become an active participant in the educational programme of the school. It will help in bringing the school and community closer. The parents who are members of the community will come to know a lot about the abilities, interests and character traits of their children through the school teachers. The parent teacher association will also enable the teachers to understand the needs of community in general. It will also provide a chance to parents to recognise the work going on in school.

(b) Inviting Distinguished Persons to School

Many a members of the community are engaged in various useful professions. They can be invited to school from time to time to share their experiences with the students. In the list of such distinguished persons the names of Sarpanch, Municipal Commissioner, Engineer, Doctor, Social Worker, Educationist, News Editors, Artisan, etc. may be included.

(c) Social Service Activities

Various social service activities can be undertaken to bring school and community closer to each other. These may include such activities as setting up of an adult education centre in school, setting up a bulletin-board and putting up on it the daily news and other useful information about the local community in particular. The members of the community can be allowed to make use of the school library and other facilities available in the school such as play grounds, gymnasium etc. The schools can also come forward to establish a first-aid post for the benefit of the community.

(d) Celebration of Festivals

School can take the lead in celebration of various festivals such as Dusherra, Diwali, Holi, Independence Day, Republic Day etc. On all such celebration the local residents be invited and may be encouraged to participate. Some type of competitions can also be arranged in the school and notable persons from the community be asked to preside over and give away prizes to the winners.

(e) Arranging Talks on National and International Topics

Talks on National and International topics may be arranged in school. To deliver such a talk some eminent member from the society be invited. The invitation to, selected few from the community be extended to attend to such a talk.

All these activities will help a lot in bringing the school and community closer to each other.

8.6. ADVANTAGES OF UTILIZING COMMUNITY RESOURCES IN SOCIAL STUDIES

Some of the advantages of utilizing community resources in Social Studies are as follows:

1. A Natural Way of Imparting Education

The survey of the community is a natural way of imparting education to the child. In it the maxim "known to unknown" works. It helps in establishing a close relationship between the child and the community.

2. Opportunities for New Interest

During survey of the community the child undertakes the study of its problems. Such a study provides to child the opportunity for the growth of new interests. Such interests are natural and creative and are not imposed from outside. They develop from within.

3. Opportunities for the Choice of the Vocation

Study of community provides the child an opportunity to choose his vocation. He observes different groups of people in the community engaged in various activities and from these observations he may be encouraged to explore his chances in industries, means of transport etc.

Such an interest will be quite helpful to the child to select a vocation of his choice.

4. Right use of Leisure

If a student becomes interested in something useful outside his school then he would spend his leisure time in that activity which may be useful to the community. It helps to develop the creativity in the child.

5. Development of Skills and Attitudes

An intimate knowledge of certain problems being faced by his community will compel him to think of plans for the development of one's city, town, country. It will help the student to become a useful citizen. It will inculcate the feeling of friendship and cooperation in the child. A pupil also gets a sense of pride by the proper study of his community. It will also arouse in him certain emotional values.

REVISION QUESTIONS

1. Write an essay on school community relationship.
2. Discuss the relationship between school and community.
3. "The school is a miniature community." Discuss.
4. Write short note on Parent-Teacher Association.
5. What are the main advantages of utilizing community resources in the teaching of Social Studies?
6. Name the important community resources and how can they be utilized in teaching of Social Studies?

9

Importance of Library in Social Studies Teaching

9.1 INTRODUCTION

These days the library is one of the important centre of resources for teaching of Social Studies. The aim of education is to train the pupils to think and form independent judgements and for attaining this aim students should be provided a variety of material. Library helps in providing this variety of material to the pupils. Library provides guidance to teacher in curriculum construction and in the selection of books. The Social Studies teacher should not follow only the text-book and he must study some standard books from the library. It will provide him a deeper understanding of the subject and a thorough command of the same. The teacher will be able to plan and organise his lesson in a better way, better than that given in the text-books.

Library is quite useful to students. When students read or consult some books from the library, their doubts become clear. Moreover the study of library books acquaint them with new exercises or problems and prepares them better for the examination. A good library also helps in inculcating proper attitudes, interests and appreciations in students. It can acquaint them with historical background of different topics and the contribution of various personalities. The library is a democratic society like ours, also fulfils its function by laying the foundation for free enquiry and intellectual development, so essential for sharing public opinion.

9.2 LIBRARY FACILITIES IN SCHOOLS

In our schools there are two types of libraries:

(a) General School Library; and

(b) Departmental Library.

(A) General School Library

In most of our schools there is a general school library which contains books and magazines on all subjects. Then there should be separate sections for history books. For the teachers there should be good books on methodology of teaching, contributions of various historians and important historical personalities. For students there should be books on recreational activities, well selected text-books, some reference books and other historical books.

Functions of School Library

Some of the important functions of school library are as follows:

1. ***It provides the Material for Instructions and Reading***

In library we have a wide variety of books including text-books and reference books and these provide the material for instruction to the teacher and a lot of reading material to the pupils. This material helps the students in completing their assignments, solving problems and doing their home task etc.

2. ***It stimulates Reading for Enjoyment and Recreation***

In the school library we find a number of books which are of general interest, both to the teacher and the pupils. In this category we include the books on travels, adventures, inventions, discoveries, biographies, story books etc. These books stimulate the teacher as well as the students to read such books first for the sake of enjoyment and recreation. In this way library helps in developing effective reading skills in the pupils.

3. ***It teaches the Technique of using the Library***

Each library follows certain rules in maintaining its books, periodicals etc. It helps to allow a proper use of the material available in the library. A definite procedure is followed to make purchases for the library, storing of books, issue of books, return of books etc. These rules are to be followed by all the members making use of the library. It helps to inculcate a definite discipline in the pupils.

4. *It provides Opportunities to Pupils to assume Responsibilities*

Library also provides various opportunities to the students as some of them may be required to help the librarian and act as library attendants or to perform various other jobs to help the librarian. While performing these jobs the pupils learn to work in co-operation, learn how to select books and so can help others in selection of books etc. All this provides to pupils an insight into human relationships, help them in understanding economic efficiency and also enables them to take action as responsible citizens whenever the occasion demands.

(B) Department Library

If resources permit a separate library be maintained for social studies. It may be housed in the social studies room. The librarian or incharge person of this library should classify the books so that students do not face any difficulty in getting the books issued. The Social Studies teacher himself should remain in touch with latest books and magazines on the subject and make additions in the library. A number of copies of good books should be purchased. A few copies of the prescribed text books be purchased for the use of poor students.

9.3 LIBRARY AS A RESOURCE CENTRE

Now-a-days when the learning process has been organised into different units of activity and experiences, the concept of library has also changed from that of a depository of books to that of a resource centre. This resource centre is most extensively used by all the members of the school family. It not only reaches every pupil and teacher of the school but also to the community in which the school is situated. It also serves as a store house of various teaching aids such as charts, maps, diagrams, pictures, models etc. In this way library can provide new depth to the learning experiences and the personal lives of the pupils. It occupies a unique position in the school. Library is a resource centre which is extensively used by all members of the school family. It helps the teacher to enrich curriculum and facilitates personal and professional reading. It helps the students to gain meaningful experiences in reading thinking and forming independent judgements. To the community, it provides for recreational and hobby interests. Library can thus justify its position as a basic tool for instructional programme. Because of the above reasons library occupies a unique position in modern school and it cannot be replaced by any other agency.

The important functions of library are:

(i) It provides material for instructions and for reading.

(ii) It stimulates reading for recreation and enjoyment.

(iii) It teaches the technique of using the library effectively.

(iv) It provides the opportunities to students to assume responsibility.

9.4. IMPORTANCE OF LIBRARY

Library has a key role in the scheme of education. Class-room teaching must be supplemented with the dissemination of knowledge through library. Different types of books in the library can be quite helpful to the students in completing the work assigned to them and to tackle all types of problems emerging from different topics prescribed in their syllabus.

Class-room teaching many a times leaves many gaps and doubts. They can be removed if students make use of good books available in the library. The teacher can help the students in the selection of good books in the library.

A library is not only a source of learning and inspiration for students but also serves the need of the teachers. A teacher must keep his knowledge ever fresh and up-to-date. This is possible by making a free use of library. He can learn latest methods of teaching from the new books available in the library. Thus a good library helps to keep the lamp of knowledge burning so as to kindle light in the minds of the students as also the teachers.

9.5 NEED FOR A SEPARATE SOCIAL STUDIES LIBRARY

The general library help in encouraging the students to make use of library services, but the students cannot get proper guidance for removing their deficiencies in a particular subject. For this a separate library for social studies is a great necessity for rendering help to the needy students. Such a library can be housed in Social Studies room and can be put under the charge of Social Studies teacher.

There should be a period of library reading in the time-table so as to enable the students of every class to make use of library. A separate social studies library is essential because of the following reasons:

(i) It helps to bring efficiency in organisation of library service.

(ii) Social studies teacher remains in constant touch with the latest books in social studies.

(iii) It provides a sense of separate identity to social studies and helps to inculcate interest in the subject.

(iv) The students get better library facilities.

(v) It helps the activities of social studies club.

(vi) It can be of a help to gifted and bright students.

Thus, it is essential that all out efforts be made to establish a separate social studies library in every school.

9.6 MATERIALS FOR SOCIAL STUDIES LIBRARY

Social studies library should contain useful audio-visual aids required for teaching of social studies. The educational pictures, charts, maps, posters about social studies be displayed on the walls of library room.

In Social studies library there should be a good collection of social studies books. The teacher should be responsible for making a wise selection of books for the library. These books should be of the following types:

(A) Book Resources

1. Text-books

A number of good text-books on various topics of Social Studies as also history of the world and history of other important countries, must be made available in the library. It is also very important to note that keeping in view in the excavations in different parts of our country and also in other parts of the world and because of rapidly changing human life in the modern age, new and revised editions of standard text-books should continually be purchased for the school library, with a view to supply up-to-date knowledge and information to teachers and students.

2. Reference Materials

These include reference books, encyclopaedias, dictionaries, year books, biographies, atlases, bibliographies, directories, old manuscripts, old coins and other excavated material, Govt. Gazetteers and the like.

3. Literary Materials

These include biographies, autobiographies, fiction, folklore, short-stories, travel books, books of adventure, hero-stories, romance, drama and poetry. This type of material provides reading for enjoyment and pleasure.

4. Source Materials

These include source books, manuscripts, original accounts of travellers and contemporary historian diaries, proclamations, original letters and dispatches of kings governors and viceroys, treaties, old monuments, historical buildings, sites, old tools, weapons, armours, coins etc.

(B) Non-Book Resources

In addition to the book resources (stated earlier) a good Social Studies library be supplemented by periodicals, pamphlets, newspapers, magazines etc. This material can be easily and inexpensively used as teaching aid in the teaching of history.

Some of the Non-Book resources available in the library are as follows:

1. Periodicals

In periodicals we include all the current event periodicals, magazines depicting different aspects of Indian life etc.

2. Pamphlets

Pamphlets are generally written about one specific topic and in most of the cases they are illustrated with pictures, photographs and drawings. Most of these are published by government agencies and bureaus for specialised services. They are quite cheap. They are very important source of information about different walks of our social, economic and political life. It is essential for a good social studies teacher to keep himself in touch with currently published pamphlets, concerning his subject.

3. Newspapers

A school should arrange to have as many newspapers as it can afford. A local newspaper is a must for every school library. In such a newspaper the students will find a number of local events, happenings, issues, developments, personalities which are correlated with the immediate social and physical environment of the child. If possible students should also procure a copy of the national dailies. A good newspaper provides at a glance the events of the world and its study is essential for the teachers and the students so that they remain in touch with the latest in the world.

4. Special Documents and Publications etc.

Most of the state governments in India publish brochures, yearly calendars or data books or activities within the states. Important business concerns, railways and tourist bureaus also publish folders, containing rich information about various places, regions and towns. The library's collection of such publications can be a valuable resource of primary source materials.

5. Audio-visual or Non-reading Materials

In addition to books, periodicals, and publications, a school library should also house a large variety of non-reading materials. Among the important visual materials we may have pictures, photographs, illustrations, maps, globes, charts, cartoons, posters, graphs, models, specimens, films-strips, slides, museum cases and display cases. Among the important auditory materials we may include radio, tape-recording, television and sound films. Auditory and visual equipment, like projectors, recorders, radio and television receivers etc. may also be housed in the library for use by the entire school. Non-reading materials play a very important part in Social Studies programme. Many of these materials present information which is difficult to obtain through reading. They add realism and furnish the class with a common background of experience.

9.7 THE SCHOOL LIBRARIAN AS A RESOURCE PERSON

A trained librarian is required in every school library for maintaining this important resource centre and to provide planned, expert service and guidance to teachers and students. However, in most of our elementary and secondary schools we have no separate librarian to play this important role. Mostly, one of the teachers is assigned this extra duty of opening the library room once or twice a week at fixed hours, to issue and receive library books. Such an arrangement defeats the very purpose for which a library is maintained in schools. It is essential that at least one full-time librarian, with a permanent assistant, be provided to every secondary school. They should also be given a separate work-room and adequate office space so as to function effectively.

A whole time trained librarian will create an atmosphere of friendliness, self-control and self-direction. He will help the students in acquiring good study habits and in developing in them a love of good books. He will also work with teachers in the proper uses of library, as an important resource centre and as a living agency. He will make available the needed resource materials to Social Studies classes because he is acquainted with all such sources.

9.8 COLLATERAL READING AND THE LIBRARY

Collateral and supplementary reading is also an essential part of Social Studies programme. In Social Studies students must collect a lot of information about various facts and movements. It is possible only after consulting many books and periodicals, besides their text-books for solving problems, doing assignments and participating in discussion etc. For this purpose library resource can provide a rich supply of books, periodicals and pamphlets for collateral reading. Text-book material must be supplemented by additional reference reading. Thus students should be encouraged to read widely on topics of their own interest, both for the sake of information and entertainment. For this purpose they should be guided how to select, read and make use of the knowledge thus obtained. In this way they will be able to form good reading habits along with proper study procedures. Students should also be encouraged to take notes and to keep a regular record of their readings.

9.9 HOW TO MOTIVATE PUPILS TO UTILIZE LIBRARY RESOURCES

In the beginning of the year, minimum amount of supplementary reading should be fixed by the teacher for each pupil. It may be different for different classes, according to their standard. Even in case of bright students and poor readers lists of different types of books, both fiction and non-fiction, especially connected with Social Studies instruction, should be prepared by the teacher in consultation with the librarian. These lists should be provided to all pupils and they may be asked to read the required number of books, out of which not more than half may be fiction.

To motivate pupils to read, the teacher should set apart some marks in this subject for supplementary reading of this type. They may be added to the total number of marks, the child receives in Social Studies at the end of the session. In this way the pupils will definitely be motivated to read.

Moreover, at the time of periodical or monthly tests, at least one question out of supplementary readers with adequate choice for different categories of pupils, should be given in the question paper, and it must be attempted compulsorily. Such a programme should, however, be made known to pupils before hand.

Further, the teacher while teaching a certain unit about a particular period in Social Studies, should bring with him such books as contain interesting accounts of living conditions in those days and read out a few paragraphs in the class from those books. He should, then, give to his pupils the names of the books, the names of the authors and those of their publishers and ask them to collect material therefrom, connected with the unit under study. After a day or two he may ask a pupil who has gone through a certain book and prepared reports and notes, to stand up and read out what be has collected pertaining to the lesson in hand. In his way, students can be motivated to read library books.

Pupils may be asked to collect from different writers, the different view points on a single topic. This is very important because instead of relying on any one source, the pupils are encouraged to draw upon several sources of information. This is perhaps the most valuable lesson that can be learnt in the library.

Teacher's Duty in the Motivation Programme

The teacher will be able to motivate his pupils for extra reading if he himself is a wide reader and is familiar with all the books published in his field. He should see that all those books are made available to students from the school library. In addition to books, he should also be a regular reader of newspapers and periodicals. The present day emphasis on current events in the teaching of Social Studies demands a good selection of newspapers and magazines for the school library. Pupils can only of encouraged to make use of this material if the teacher has himself formed a habit of reading a daily newspaper and at least one or two magazines, related to history and making current-events a basis of study of some important unit in Social Studies.

Teacher should also keep a record of the library study of each student as it may help him in evaluating a student's performance.

REVISION QUESTIONS

1. What are the important functions of a library?
2. What are the different library resources for teaching Social Studies?
3. How can a social studies teacher encourage his students to read?
4. What should be the essential equipments for a school library?
5. How can the teacher motivate his students to read library books?

10

Social Studies Text-book

10.1 INTRODUCTION

Text-books are standardized collection of the subject-matter that has to be taught to the students. They facilitate the teaching of new concepts and skills and maintain knowledge already acquired and help the correlation of the theoretical knowledge with the practical aspects of life. There are three categories of text-books:

(i) Reference books

(ii) Main text-books, and

(iii) Supplementary books.

10.2 IMPORTANCE OF TEXT-BOOKS

Before script came into existence and press came into being, most of the education was imparted orally and verbally. This tradition was all the more prevalent in India. It was at a very late stage that text-books came to be used in education. In the western world, it was after French Revolution that text-books came to be used in education. Later on in America this device was employed. Since then they are being used. In India the text-books were used after script came into existence and the verbal knowledge was transcribed on the leaves of the trees. In the Islamic world, Holy Quran formed the text-book of the earliest education of the child. This was also a written book.

Text-books have an importance in the field of education. They are a device of imparting knowledge to the students. They save a lot of time and economise the human labour. H.R. Douglus has rightly said that, "In the last analysis with the great majority of the teachers, the text-book is potent determinant of what and how they will teach.

The teacher is the workman, who moulds the lives of the students into various forms. He has to use the text-books as the instruments. If the instruments are not good the workman shall not be able to present his best. Similarly, if the text-books are not good, the teacher is not able to present the best before the students. Raymont has rightly said:

> "The text-book must be regarded as strictly subordinate and supplementary to the teacher lesson."

10.3 VALUE OF GOOD TEXT-BOOK

The value of a good text-book of Social Studies is considered under various headings:

(a) Utility to the teacher.

(b) Utility to the student.

(c) Utility to maintain uniform standards.

Utility of Text-books in the Teaching of Social Studies

A great deal of controversy exists about the utility of text-books in the teaching of social studies. Some educationists have opined that text-books should not be used at all while others are of the opinion that the text-books should form the real base of education. Both these opinions are the extremes. Actually the best way is to strike a balance between the two. Text-books should be used in teaching of Social Studies but they should be used economically. They should be used to help the students to strengthen their experiences or to help the students to revise their lessons which they have learnt in the classroom. Text-books can also be used by the students to write down the answers to the questions that the teacher asks them to write down.

Text-books should serve as tools in the hands of the teachers. They should help the teachers to make their teaching more authentic, successful and effective. Earnest Horne has rightly remarked:

> "One of the most effective ways for improving the content and method of instruction is to place better text-books in the hands of teachers and pupils."

In this regards Prof. Hardikar says, "The text-book is a totality of items of knowledge, habits, feelings, activities and attitudes."

A. Utility to the Teacher

(i) It provides suitable subject-matter and guidelines regarding the syllabus of the subject. So the teacher neglects no portion of the syllabus and does not waste time on irrelevant details.

(ii) It helps the teacher to teach in an organised and systematic way, as it contains various topics in a proper sequence.

(iii) It is the most reliable source of information as it is generally written by experienced teachers. It serves as a reference book to the teacher.

(iv) A good text-book suggests the steps of planning, method of teaching and suitable illustrative materials to the teacher, regarding a particular topic.

(v) It provides certain well-illustrated examples about a topic.

(vi) It provides the teacher with a number of well-graded problems which he can give to the students.

(vii) Text-books help the teacher in assigning home-work to his students. They also help him to assign drill work.

(viii) It also suggests possibilities of correlation and related project activities.

B. Utility to the Students

Text-books are quite useful from the point of view of students as they save their time and they are saved from taking class notes.

Some other uses are:

(i) They provide the students with well-graded exercises for drill, revision and review.

(ii) Text-books help a student to understand the subject-matter as it makes the things clear.

(iii) Since every text-book contains some solved problems so the student can take help of these problems in solving other unsolved problems.

(iv) The student can learn a topic in advance with the help of text-book.

(v) Text-books are also quite useful in case a student has to remain absent from class due to one or the other reason.

C. Utility to Maintain Uniform Standards

Text-books play an important role in maintaining a uniformity in standards. The text-books are quite helpful to examiners in their evaluation work because they come to know of the standards expected of a particular class.

10.4 CHARACTERISTICS OF A GOOD TEXT-BOOK

The text-book helps the teacher to know what he has to teach; it helps the students to revise what has been taught to them in the classroom. Only a good text-book will help in this matter. The selection of a good text-book has to be done by the teacher. The teacher should keep the following points in mind while making such a selection:

1. It presents the subject-matter strictly in accordance with the latest syllabus.
2. It is written by experienced teachers.
3. It is written according to the aims and objectives of teaching of social studies.
4. It presents the subject-matter in a proper sequence. It may be so organised that it may be possible for the students to revise what they have learnt in the class. An effort be made to present the topic in a spiral form.
5. It should contain well-graded problems for revision.
6. The books be so written that they awaken intellectual curiosity of the students and also keeps their interest alive.
7. The language of the book should be in accordance with the age group of the students.
8. The printing and get up of the book should be attractive.
9. It should suggest the teaching method, the possible aids for teaching the topic, correlation of the topic and the activities or practical work connected with the topic.
10. It should contain well-illustrated material but not too many solved problems. The answers given to problems should be correct.
11. It must also contain objective type and short answer questions.

12. Hints for difficult problems be provided.
13. It should be moderately priced.
14. It should give only up-to-date material.

Thus to evaluate a Social Studies text-book, the criterion may be useful content material, proper organisation of subject-matter, proper gradation of the exercises, material aid devices for motivation, simple language, good number of illustrations, good printing and an impressive get up. It should be moderately priced and free from mistakes and errors. It should not contain too many solved problems and should be up-to-date in its contents.

10.5 TASK OF WRITING TEXT-BOOKS

To write a text-book is not an easy task. Text-books must be planned in a scientific way and the subject-matter be presented in a psychological way. Text-book should not only present the subject-matter but should present it in a manner suitable for the students. The subject-matter be arranged to meet the requirements of the age and stage of the students. The various qualities of good text-books have already been discussed and these qualities must be found in good text-books.

10.6 TEXT-BOOKS OF SOCIAL STUDIES FOR VARIOUS STAGES OF EDUCATION

The various stages of education are:

1. Primary
2. Junior High School
3. Secondary, and
4. Higher.

In the present chapter, we are not concerned with the text-books of pre-primary and higher stages of education. We are primarily concerned with the text-books to be used in the Primary, Junior High School and Secondary classes. Text-books meant for these various stages of education should have certain qualities and requisites as laid down below:

(i) **Text-books of Civics for Primary Classes:** Here the students upto the age of 11 come to receive education. Such children are very fond of listening to stories. Curiosity is their basic instinct. Text-books that are intended for this stage of education, should have the following qualities in them:

1. The subject-matter should be presented in form of a story.
2. Books should be profusely illustrated. There should be a good deal of charts and pictures.
3. They should be written in a simple language and lucid style. This would enable the students to understand the subject-matter easily and quickly.
4. The text-book should be written with an eye on the psychological requirements of the children of this age.
5. These books should not be very bulky.
6. The subject-matter of the book should be based on the principle of selectivity. Such subject-matter should find a place in these text-books that shall be useful for developing certain requisite qualities in the children of this age group.
7. The book should be perfectly in accordance with the syllabus and the curriculum laid down for this stage of education.
8. The title cover should be very attractive so that it may catch the eyes of the students at the first glance.
9. Books should be reasonably priced. These should not cost too much as to be beyond the reach of the common man.
10. They should intend at inculcating social qualities in the students.
11. The main aim of teaching Social Studies is to produce ideal citizens of the country. The seeds for ideal citizenship should be shown at this stage of education, with the help of these text-books.

Activity and creativity should be developed in the students with the help of these text-books. In other words, it means that the subject-matter should be so presented that there may be a good deal of scope for creative activities in the students.

(ii) **Text-books of Social Studies for the Students of Junior High School Classes:** At this stage of education students between the age group of 11 and 14 are found. These students are on the gateway of adolescence. They do not take interest in listening to stories only. They want to face the realities of life to some extent. Text-books of Social Studies intended for the students of this stage of education, should be written in more or less narrative style. They, in order to be useful, should have the following qualities:

1. Text-books of Social Studies for this stage of education should be written with an eye on the mental and the physical age of the students. They should keep in view the interest, aptitudes and talents of the student.
2. The subject-matter should be properly graded.
3. At the end of each chapter there should be certain questions for recapitulation.
4. The printing and the get up of the text-book should be flawless and attractive.
5. There should be charts, pictures, illustrations, etc. These charts and illustrations should be attractive, precise and neatly drawn.
6. The text-books should form to the aims and objectives of the teaching of Social Studies at this stage of education.
7. They should also develop the qualities of ideal citizenship in the students.
8. An attempt should also be made to develop the social qualities in the students.
9. Social Studies is a subject which requires more of practical training than theoretical teaching. Text-books should aim at this objective. This training has to begin at the Junior High School stage of education.

(iii) **Text-books for Secondary Classes of Education:** This is the stage of adolescence. Students between 14-18 years of age come and receive education at this level. They are interested in taking a practical view of life. They want to solve problems by themselves. Their curiosity of listening to stories has come to an end. Certain other instincts and tendencies start developing by now. The text-books in order to be useful and successful, should cater to these psychological needs. They should have the following characteristics as well:

1. Firstly, they should be different from the text-books intended for the students of the Primary and the Junior High

School classes. There is little scope for story telling and dialogues at this stage of education. There should be narration of facts. This narration should be of a realistic nature but interesting.

2. The subject-matter of the text-books should be so organised that it may satisfy the mental faculties of thinking, reasoning, imagination etc.
3. The subject-matter should be properly selected. It should be so selected as to meet the requirements of the psychological needs of this stage of education.

Problems of social, political and moral value should form the subject-matter of teaching at this stage of education. It is natural for text-books to present these problems in an interesting and effective manner.

4. Students of this age are fond of solving the problems. Various problems concerning civic life should be so presented before the students, of course, through text-books, that they may take an active part in them and try to solve those problems.
5. Text-books of social studies for the students of Higher Secondary classes should have a good number of graphs and charts in them. These graphs and charts are helpful in encouraging the students to take up serious study of Social Studies.
6. There is scope for giving facts and figures in the text-books meant for this stage of education. These facts and figures should be recent ones.
7. The language and the style of the text-books of this stage of education has a specific importance. The style should be lucid, no doubt, but it should be well-polished. The language should be easy but it should be able to convey the thoughts properly and effectively. The subject-matter should be properly organised and categorised. The sequence of the sentence should not be very complex. In short, an attempt should be made to present the subject-matter in an attractive and effective manner.
8. The subject-matter of the text-books should be properly correlated. An attempt should be made to correlate the subject-

matter of social studies with that of history, political science and such other social science that have a direct bearing on the subject-matter of Social Studies.

9. Since the subject-matter of Social Studies is more of a practical nature, an attempt should be made to employ Project Method, Problem Method, Activity Method, Excursion Method etc. in its teaching. An attempt should be made to reflect these methods in text-books as well.
10. Subject-matter of Social Studies is of a changing nature. Every year we find some changes in the structure of the administration or the working of the civic life. The text-books should be kept up-to-date.
11. The text-books for this stage of education should be reasonably priced.
12. At the end of every chapter, there should be a set of questions. These questions should be psychologically planned and scientifically presented. They should help the recapitulation of the subject proves taught.

In short, the text-books should meet all the requirements of this stage of education. Text-books of Social Studies are not very up-to-date. Following extract from Secondary Education Commission Report proves this point further:

"We are greatly dissatisfied with the present standard of production of school books and consider it essential that it should be radically improved."

10.7 NEEDS AND PLACE OF A SOCIAL STUDIES TEXT-BOOK

What is the place for the text-book in modern education? At present the essence of teaching consists in helping the child to discover things for himself. But this is not all. We should proceed from the concrete to the abstract. But we must not remain in the abstract; we should come back again to the concrete. Knowledge is power only when it is used and for using it we require assimilation which comes from drill and discipline. In high and higher secondary classes, teaching does not and should not end with the class-period. Knowledge is not only to be experienced and discovered, but also remembered and applied. For achieving this end, a complete record of class-notes must be kept. However, our average school-pupils cannot be expected to listen, understand and take down notes simultaneously. Therefore the teacher has to give notes and problems for exercise. A good teacher will certainly like to draw up his own scheme of studies as well as notes and exercises. But every teacher is not expected to be equal to the task nor our education system allows him this freedom. It is here that the need of a good-book arises in teaching a subject like Social Studies.

Moreover, Social Studies is a new subject in the curriculum. Suitable text-books on this subject are not yet available in good number. The result is that at the initial stages either separate books written on history, geography and civics are being used or bulky volume of books on Social Studies containing topics from history, geography and civics combined together. But such books are of little use because they are not written according to the true concept of Social Studies. Authors of such books have never thought that Social Studies is a compact whole whose object is to adjust the students to their social environment (which includes the family, community, state and nation) so that they may be able to understand how society has come to its present form and how to interpret intelligently the matrix of social forces and movements in the midst of which they are living. So the Social Studies teachers are grouping their way in the dark. For their guidance, good text-books on Social Studies, written round topics, themes, movements or problems, are essential. For some time the chief basis of Social Studies instruction has to be the text-book, written according to the concept, aims and objectives of this new subject. If we really wish that its teaching is not strange in its infancy, we should produce and use really good text-books on Social Studies.

10.8 HOW TO USE A TEXT-BOOK?

It is generally seen that most of the students and teachers in India regard the text-book as a very simple device. They assume that all its aspects and features are self-explanatory and they can secure all its advantages without experience, application or special training. They are wrong in their assumption. In fact, the text-book is a very compact and somewhat complicated product. As such its correct use requires considerable understanding and skill. Some of its most helpful features, require explanation and drill if they are to yield the maximum values. Since a lot of time and attention are devoted to a text-book, the teacher should see that students learn how to utilize it most profitably. Better if the teacher could occasionally give a demonstration in the right use of a text-book along with his comments and then ask his pupils to follow in that manner. It should be remembered that text-book is not a method of teaching. It is only an effective device of teaching.

The following suggestions are given for the effective use of a Social Studies text-book:

1. **Introduction of its contents.** In the beginning of the year pupils should be introduced to the contents of the entire book, along with its special features. This will help them in getting an idea of the complete programme of Social Studies and build up a general readiness for the work of the entire year.
2. **Determining the sequence of contents.** The author of the text-book may have written it strictly in accordance with the prescribed syllabus, without caring for the logical arrangement of the subject-matter. He is not in a position to judge all the factors which suit best a particular class, at a particular place. It is, therefore, essential that the teacher should determine the sequence of contents that will suit best his purpose in the beginning of the year.
3. **Developing a readiness for each unit.** This involves some class discussion, map work, story telling or similar activities, which "set the stage" for the main part of the unit, to be undertaken.
4. **Proper use of questions and exercises at the end of the unit.** The text-book exercises, given at the end of each unit or chapter, should be studied by the teacher before-hand to determine with best possible use. These can be used for providing more challenging work to one or two selected groups of pupils and for revision work for the rest of the class.

In short Social Studies text-book should be used to stimulate a spirit of further enquiry, in accordance with the abilities and interests of the pupils and to some extent, according to availability of sources.

REVISION QUESTIONS

1. Bring out the importance of text-books in teaching Social Studies.
2. What is the utility of text-books in teaching of Social Studies?
3. What are the characteristics of good text-book?
4. What are the good ways of using a text-book?
5. Discuss the essential qualities of a good text-book on Social Studies.

11

Social Studies Room or Laboratory

11.1 INTRODUCTION

Like any other subject rooms there should be a separate room for Social Studies. The setting and arrangement of this room should be such that it creates an atmosphere for the study and teaching of Social Studies. The students entering the room would find themselves interested in the learning of Social Studies.

At present we have various types of teaching aids such as text-books, reference books, pamphlets, maps, charts, projectors, models, magazines etc. and these can be properly used if they are stored in a systematic way in a separate room called the Social Studies room. In fact a well equipped social studies room is essential for fostering a particular attitude of mind among the pupils.

It has been observed by M.P. Mofatt, "Classroom furnishing and their arrangements have direct bearing upon the quality of results obtained. Satisfactory outcomes can be expected from any class-room situation only when adequate facilities are provided. It should be furnished to provide a suitable environment for acquiring and practicing social studies skills."

A provision of a special room for Social Studies is desirable because of the following considerations:

(i) Providing 'home of their own' to teachers for developing enthusiasm for the subject and faith in themselves and students.

(ii) Creating and maintaining an effective teaching-learning environment.

(iii) Providing a quick and ready functional environment by making available work-room for the students.

(iv) Introducing variety in teaching methods and facilitating the use of teaching aids readily and conveniently.

(v) Saving energy and time in carrying round equipment like charts, maps, models, pictures and projectors etc.

11.2 NEED OF A SOCIAL STUDIES LABORATORY

As we need a laboratory to teach physical sciences such as physics, chemistry or life sciences such as botany, zoology etc., so also we need a laboratory to teach social studies which is a social science. In the laboratory of social studies the students will undertake various types of activities such as research, construction, music, dramatic and creative art etc. in a free and desirable environment.

With the drastic changes that have taken place in educational methodology whereby teachers have become more and more concerned with the physical facilities to accomplish the good work. He is now highly dependent on different types of teaching aids such as text-books, pamphlets, magazines, maps, globes, charts etc. It is, therefore, that educators today, have realised the necessity to have a separate social studies laboratory or a room wherein such an environment prevails that promote an excellent teaching process. Such a class-room, with a pleasant social climate, becomes a learning laboratory in which great emphasis is put on students activity and student participation in class-room procedures. In such a class-room students feel at home and quite comfortable and have an incentive to work, "class-room furnishing and their arrangement have direct bearing upon the quality of results obtained. Satisfactory outcomes can be expected from any class-room situation only when adequate and comfortable working facilities are provided. It is furnished to provide a suitable environment for acquiring and practising social studies."

With new method of teaching a need is felt more and more to have a room with special setting, where all the essential equipment for teaching are easily accessible. Hence, the need for a separate social studies class-room or laboratory.

11.3 EQUIPMENT OF THE SOCIAL STUDIES ROOMS

It should be provided with the following equipments:

1. Audio-visual material including film strip, epidiascope, projector, magic lantern, tape recorder etc.

2. Bulleting-boards
3. Charts and graphs
4. Globes
5. Maps and Atlases
6. Flags
7. Models
8. Some meteorological instruments such as barometer, rain guage etc.
9. Rocks and minerals
10. Stamps.
11. Survey instruments such as compass, chain, arrows, divider, scale etc.
12. Slide album containing slides showing architecture, dancing, music, painting etc.
13. Time charts and graphs.
14. Text-books
15. Reference books
16. Unit booklets dealing with different topics
17. Literary material
18. Periodicals and magazines
19. Newspapers
20. Pamphlets published by various agencies including central and state governments and also agencies such as UNO, UNESCO etc.

The utility of these items is given in brief:

I. Chalk Board

The colour of such a board may be green, yellow, white or even black. This is used to draw outline pictures as also to write summaries etc. It should be located at such a place that it can easily be seen by the students.

II. Bulletin-board

It is used to display maps, charts, current events, news-items, paper cuttings, magazine articles etc.

III. Furniture

Sufficient furniture for sitting of the students be provided. It should also be provided with a movable desk or table and a chair for the teacher. In addition to this it should be provided with a table dictionary, desk calender, pen, etc., for teachers use.

IV. Books and Book Cases

Text-books by different authors, current magazines, periodicals, reference books be provided in sufficient numbers so that students have an easy access to the reading material. Open-book shelves may be provided for storing these items.

V. Audio-visual Teaching Aids

The Social Studies room should be fully equipped with various types of audio-visual teaching aids such as pictures, maps, models, specimens, films, film-strips, globe etc. If possible provision should also be made to have projectors, record player, radio-set and tape recorder in the social studies room. These teaching aids play an important role in teaching of social studies.

VI. Collections

A corner in the social studies room be reserved for old coins, old clothes, dresses, utencils, historical relics, old paintings, art pictures etc. Such items may be got collected through social studies students.

Flags of different nations be also exhibited in the social studies room. It need be a brief history of such flags may also be tagged with the flags.

VII. Paints, Water Colours etc.

Social studies room should also be provided with paints, water colours, coloured pencils, inks, pen-holders, brushes, rulers, compasses, erasers, scissors, blotters, special papers of different size and colour, paste, paper clips, drawing set, pins, nails etc. All these things are needed by students for their practical work in social studies.

VIII. Cabinets and Files

Cabinets and files are required to store different materials. The filing system is helpful in locating the needed article at once.

The above points can be summarised as under:

(a) It should be spacious enough as to accommodate the students and have space for demonstrations, models, black-board and charts etc.

(b) It should also have arrangement for acting certain dramas.

(c) There should be a good arrangement of black-boards. Teaching of social studies requires a lot of use of black-boards. There may be overlapping boards. Such arrangement would facilitate the drawing of charts and the maps.

(d) There should be a small collection of books in the social studies room.

(e) The social studies room should be decorated with the pictures of historical personalities and charts etc. There should also be pictures of the battles and wars and similar events.

(f) There should be arrangement of Epidiascope. There should also be arrangement of globes and project pictures.

11.4 ADVANTAGES OF SOCIAL STUDIES ROOM

Various advantages of a separate social studies room for the teaching of stocial studies as under:

1. **Scientific Teaching**. It helps to make it possible to bring about the scientific teaching of the subject.
2. **It makes Teaching of Social Studies Effective.** In the absence of a separate social studies room, the teacher has to carry the teaching aids and other materials with him. Such steps are not needed when there is a separate social studies room. It saves the spoiling of the material for the teaching of social studies, in the transit and also the time.
3. **Proper Atmosphere**. It creates an atmosphere suitable and congenial for the teaching of social studies.
4. **It develops the Power of Imagination and Observation.** In a particularly equipped social studies room, there are maps, charts and other useful things for the teaching of social studies. These things help to develop power of observation and imagination of the students.

All these things are possible if the social studies room is properly equipped.

11.5 CLASS-ROOM MANAGEMENT

The social studies room should be the place where a healthy social relationship develops between pupils and pupils and also between teacher and pupils. To achieve it students be given their due share in the management of the social studies room. Various committees be formed for purchase, collection, arrangement etc., and students be given a training for group leadership and committee co-operation through such committees.

In the words of Moffatt and Howell "Class-room management expresses a business-like and orderly approach to the teaching-learning situation. Leadership gives direction and provides for the type of atmosphere so essential for effective instruction. Good organisation for all activities eliminates confusion and possible discipline problems. Pupils should, therefore, be encouraged to develop abilities and attitude commensurate with the democratic sharing of responsibilities in the co-management of their own class-room." Good work should be appreciated and each student should be encouraged to show his worth. Opportunities for self-discipline and self-control, based on co-operation, should be provided to all pupils. This will lead to character building and personal development. If our students assume responsibilities in the true spirit and discharge them to the best of their abilities and capacities, they are receiving effective training for democratic citizenship.

11.6 LABORATORY-WORK IN SOCIAL STUDIES

Besides regular social studies periods provided in the school time-table, some periods be allotted for *laboratory work* in social studies. The basic purpose of laboratory work is to develop skills, original thinking, planning and to develop creative expression among students. In the laboratory-work period students are busy in drawing maps, preparing graphs, charts, time lines, models or pictures, solving problems, working on projects and answering given questions and assignments individually or in groups. Specific instructions are given tc students regarding the work to be done and sources from where the material is to be collected. They try to learn through research

Social Studies Laboratory

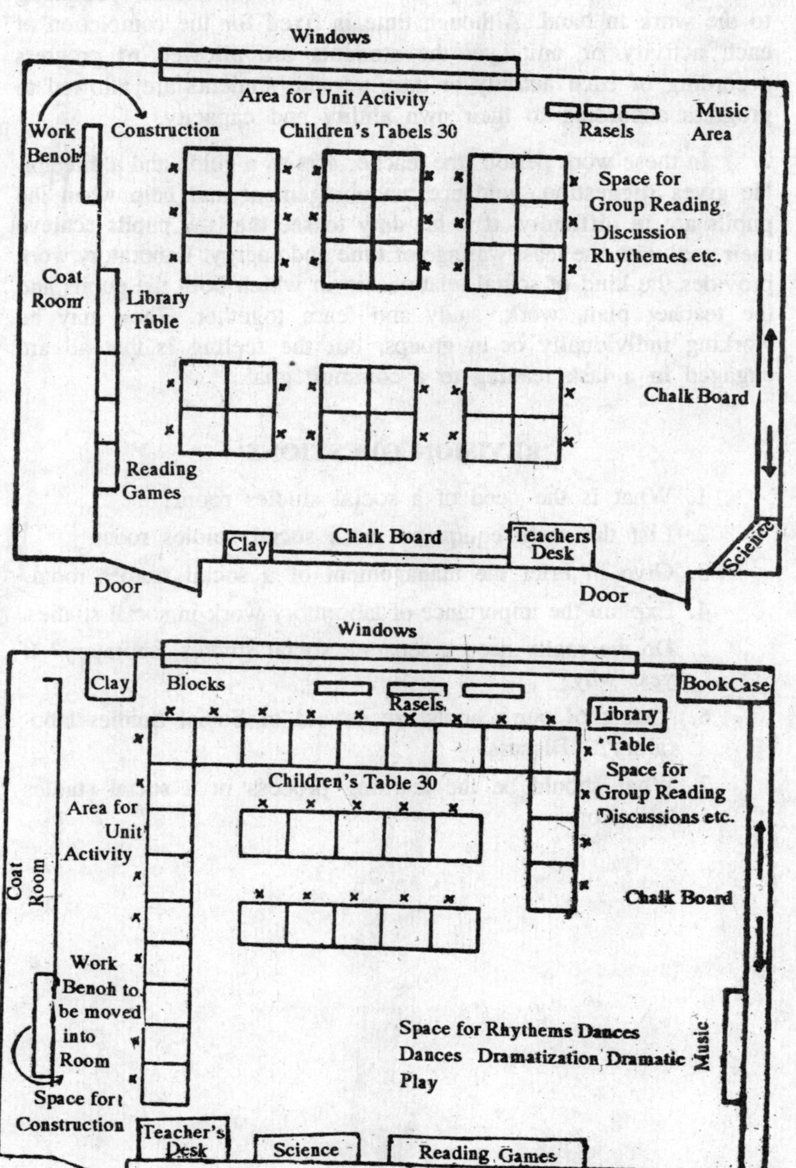

and exploration. They are given freedom to move about the classroom and make maximum possible use of the material, pertaining to the work in hand. Although time is fixed for the completion of each activity or unit, yet the students are allowed to progress according of each activity or unit, yet the students are allowed to progress according to their own ability and capacity.

In these work periods the teacher acts as a guide and a director. He gives suggestion, guidance, encouragement and help when the pupils are in difficulty. It is his duty to see that the pupils achieve their goal with the least wastage of time and energy. Laboratory work provides the kind of social relationship in which both the pupils and the teacher plan, work, study and learn together. They may be working individually or in groups, but the feeling is that all are engaged in a task leading to a common goal.

REVISION QUESTIONS

1. What is the need of a social studies room?
2. List the main equipment of a social studies room.
3. Give in brief the management of a social studies room.
4. Explain the importance of laboratory work in social studies.
5. Do we really need a separate social studies laboratory? If yes, why?
6. "Most of our schools are devoid of Social Studies laboratory? Discuss.
7. What should be the learning process in a social studies laboratory?

12

Social Studies Teacher

12.1 INTRODUCTION

The success or failure of a social studies course rests mainly with the teacher. He may be provided with all the possible facilities in terms of laboratory, apparatus and equipment, given an ideal syllabus and a sufficient time for teaching social studies but unless he is enthusiastic about his work, knows the subject and really knows how to teach social studies, he is not likely to achieve success. On the other hand a keen and well-informed teacher who loves his subject and believes in its value will succeed in spite of difficulties and handicaps.

In this regard the Kothari Commission Report (1966) says, "Of all the different factors which influence the quality of education and its contribution to national development, the quality, competence and character of teachers are undoubtedly the most significant."

Dr. S. Radhakrishnan emphasises the role of teacher in the following words, "The teacher's place in society is of vital importance. He acts as the pivot for transmission of intellectual traditions and technical skill from generation to generation, and helps to keep the lamp of civilisation burning. He not only guides the individual, but also, so to say, the destiny of nation." Teachers have therefore to realise their special responsibility to the society. On the other hand, it is incumbent on the society to pay due regard to the teaching profession and to ensure that the teacher is kept above want and given the status which will command respect from his student.

12.2 IMPORTANCE OF SOCIAL STUDIES TEACHER

Social Studies, as a subject, is a new-comer in the school ccurriculum. Only a few people understand its true nature and still fewer can teach it satisfactorily. Social Studies, more than any other subject, demands well-prepared and conscientious men and women of sound knowledge and good training. It is in this subject that in addition to the prescribed subject-matter, the teacher is also required to deal with attitudes, skills and appreciations. It is he who is expected to produce intelligent citizens and responsible leaders for the next generation. It is he who is to handle the raw human material and develop it for successful democratic living. It is his duty to transform this material into well-adjusted, well-informed and happy citizens who will participate successfully in matters of national and international importance. As such, the future of the child, the future of the school, the future of the community, the future of the nation and the future of mankind at large, depends upon the Social Studies' teacher. He is, thus, the real, "architect of nation." Perhaps H.G. wells was pointing to Social Studies teacher when he remarked: "The teacher is the real maker of history." In the school, he is a substitute of the parent; a friend, a guide and a true master. He is, in fact, the soul of the school and everything that goes about it.

12.3 PLACE OF THE TEACHER

Independent India has by common consent adopted democracy as the best form of government. Democracy however needs a body of citizens who are ever prepared to shoulder the responsibilities that go with freedom. To have such citizens tomorrow, we must develop in our children and youth of today the knowledge, competence and sense of values that would make them effective members of the nation. In this respect social studies can contribute the most. A great responsibility, therefore, devolves upon the teacher of social studies. He must thoroughly prepare to meet the challenge.

Teacher is the real source of education. Truly speaking education is a tri-polar process and consists of *child (pupil), subject-matter*, and the *teacher*, child is the focal point (central part) around which the whole process revolves. The *teacher* tries to teach the *child* the *subject-matter*. While teaching the child, the teacher has to keep an eye on the psychological requirements of the child. It is the teacher who actually guides the destiny of the child. Teacher handles the subject-matter in such a way that the students are equipped for their future life. For any nation to progress we need a team of successful teachers. If a nation has only incompetent teachers it is sure to go down.

In the words of Prof. Binning, "Teacher is the pivot around which whole educational system moves."

The teacher is like a gardner who tends the tender plants of society and help them to blossom forth into full bloom and fragrance. The teacher of social studies in this regard tries to fill the fragrance of ideal citizenship into the future flowers of civic life of the land.

12.4 ROLE OF SOCIAL STUDIES TEACHER IN THE LIFE OF THE SCHOOL

A social studies teacher is expected to play a very important role in the life of the school. Some of the roles expected of him are:

(i) Serving on school committees.
(ii) Working with parents.
(iii) Counselling students.
(iv) Filling out reports.
(v) Acting as a home room teacher or house master.
(vi) Serving on duty around the school.
(vii) Having contacts with school officials.
(viii) Issuing grades and reports.
(ix) Taking part in co-curricular activities.
(x) Working with clerical staff of the school.
(xi) Taking part in social affairs with teachers and students.
(xii) Taking part in community activities.
(xiii) Assisting student teachers.
(xiv) Participating in professional activities.
(xv) Performing miscellaneous duties in the total life of the school.

Duties of the Teacher of Social Studies

The main duties of the teacher of social studies, to inculcate in the students the values of ideal citizenship. In order to achieve this objective he has to undertake the following jobs:

(1) Teacher should act as a student. In other words, he has to study the interest, aptitudes and other mental faculties of the students and impart knowledge of social studies to them with an eye on all these mental faculties.

(2) He should keep himself up-to-date about the problems of social studies life. He should know the most recent events of civic life.

(3) No curriculum of Social Studies can be complete and up-to-date. Social Studies is an evergrowing subject. The teacher of Social Studies has act as a Curriculum Construction Expert. He has to fit in the different developments of the civic life in the curriculum in such a way that the students may not feel that he is reading something that is not of interest and of value to him.

(4) The Social Studies teacher is to act as a link between the School and the civic life at large. He has to establish cor-relationship between the life and the school and the life of various other associations and social groups. The main aim of teaching of Social Studies is to establish an ideal civic life. It is the duty of the Social Studies Teacher to encourage the students to play their role in this direction.

12.5 QUALITIES AND CHARACTERISTICS OF A SUCCESSFUL SOCIAL STUDIES TEACHER

In order to achieve the above mentioned objectives and to discharge the tasks expected of a Social Studies teacher, he should have the following qualities.

(1) Ideal citizen,

(2) Faith in the teaching of the subject and profession,

(3) Thorough knowledge of the subject,

(4) Impartiality and scientific outlook,

(5) Sympathy and creative imagination,

(6) Impressive and interesting personality,

(7) Faith in democracy,

(8) Love and affections for the students,

(9) Ideal social worker,

(10) Ideal leader, and

(11) Properly equipped.

1. Ideal Citizen

According to an old saying "Example is always better than a precept." The teacher of Social Studies has to prove this saying all the more by his actions. Social Studies has a practical aspect as well. It has to train young students to become ideal citizens. A teacher of Social Studies has to present the example of ideal citizen to be able to encourage the students to acquire the qualities of ideal citizenship.

2. Faith in the Teaching of the Subject and the Profession

The teacher of Social Studies should have faith in the profession as also the utility of teaching Social Studies to the students. Unless a person has faith in the job that is entrusted, he will not be able to do full justice to it. This faith encourages a person to acquire more and discharge his duties in an ideal manner. The teacher of Social Studies should have this faith in him.

Unless the teacher is convinced of the utility of teaching Social Studies, he shall not be able to do justice to the subject.

3. Thorough Knowledge of the Subject

The teacher should have a thorough knowledge of the subject. If he has no command over the subject he shall not able to present the subject-matter before the students in an interesting manner. The teacher of Social Studies should know the correlationship of Social Studies and Social Science. He should also be aware of the current events and duties of a citizen. He should also know where the interest of the nation lies. Unless he has all these qualities in him he shall not able to teach the students successfully.

4. Impartiality and Scientific Outlook

The teacher of Social Studies should be impartial. He should try to present the subject-matter in an objective manner. If he is not able to do that, he shall not be able to inculcate the spirit of true citizenship in the students. If the teacher colours the subject-matter with his personal views and likes and dislikes, he shall not be doing justice, either to the students or to the subject.

The presentation of the subject-matter should be systematic and proper. It can be possible only if the teacher has a scientific outlook.

5. Sympathy and Creative Imagination

The elements of sympathy enables a person to understand things properly. This quality also helps the teacher to know the viewpoints of the students. Creative imagination helps the teacher to present the subject-matter in a lively and interesting manner. Ross has remarked that the person from whom a gift of sympathy is withheld should not become teacher.

6. Impressive and Interesting Personality

Personality of the teacher plays an important role in the classroom. If the teacher has an impressive and interesting personality he is able to impress the students well. It is quite possible that a teacher may have certain drawbacks in the personality but he can overcome them by certain other accomplishments.

7. Faith in Democracy

Citizenship is very much needed for a democratic way of life. Unless the teacher has full faith in democracy and democratic way of life, it shall not be possible for him to teach social studies properly. For efficient functioning of democracy the citizens must know their rights and duties. They have to be conscious of their social obligations and needs. Only such teacher, who has full faith in democracy, can teach all these things to his students.

8. Love and Affection for the Students

The teacher of Social Studies should have a mastery of child psychology and educational psychology. Unless he has the knowledge of all these things as also the knowledge of the method of teaching and the principles and objectives of teaching, he cannot discharge his job successfully. The teacher who is endowed with all these qualities, shall have love and affection for his students. He should treat the students as if they were his own kith and kin and would treat them sympathetically. Such an atmosphere is congenial for teaching, specially for the teaching of Social Studies.

9. Ideal Social Worker

The teacher of Social Studies makes an effort to build the lives of his students. This life building can be possible only when he is intimate with the spirit of social service. Developing the students into ideal citizens is the greatest social service that can be done. The teaching of Social Studies has the practical aspect in this respect. Thus teacher of Social Studies should act as a social worker and inculcate in the students the spirit of social services and ideal citizenship.

10. Ideal Leader

The teacher of Social Studies should have the qualities of an ideal leader. A teacher who has this quality is able to impress the students more. He is able to guide the students in the proper direction. Since teaching of Social Studies has the practical aspect as well, an ideal leader can lead his followers in the right direction.

11. Properly Equipped

The teacher of Social Studies should be properly equipped. He should know the method of teaching as well as other requirements of a teacher. As already stated he should have the knowledge of child psychology as well as educational psychology. If he has these qualities he will be able to do real job. Prof. Hardikar has summed up these qualities in the following words:

> "A teacher of Social Studies must be, in short, himself a good and worthy citizen, like an American citizen in the days of Pericles. Only a citizen-teacher can induce 'civic consciousness' in his pupils."

Eight C's of an Effective Social Studies Teacher

(i) Content mastery
(ii) Confidence
(iii) Caring for the pupils

(iv) Communication skill
(v) Creativity
(vi) Curiosity
(vii) Commitment
(viii) Catalytic power.

Nine Special Qualities of a Social Studies Teachers

(i) Art of development of human relations
(ii) Objectivity
(iii) Deep knowledge of the subject
(iv) Application of field study theory
(v) A well-informed teacher
(vi) Widely travelled person
(vii) A good communicator
(viii) Skilled in the use of technological aids
(ix) An interpreter of various experiences.

12.6. SELF-APPRAISAL BY A SOCIAL STUDIES TEACHER

A Social Studies teacher may evaluate himself by taking into consideration the following points:

A. Attitude Towards the Subject

1. Does my attitude towards the teaching of social studies stress facts to the neglect of ideas?
2. Do I obtain most of my social knowledge from books?
3. Do I observe events and trends in my community with a reasonable degree of insight and critical judgement?
4. Do my assignments emphasise facts at the expense of interpretation of critical judgement?
5. Do my tests give students an opportunity to exhibit that they have passed from memorisation to such procedure as comparison, contrast, selection, evaluation, deduction and judgement?
6. Do I help my students to interpret successfully the meaning of factual material?

7. Do I help students to use terms with precision?
8. Do I try to restrain excessive use of emotion in the thought processes of students?
9. Do I encourage the students to ask questions that show the development of capacities higher than that of memory alone?
10. Do students show a capacity to apply in civics those procedures that are expected in science--collecting and cataloguing the facts and drawing conclusions from them?
11. Are students becoming increasingly aware of the importance of relevance in the discussion of a subject?
12. Am I constantly relating social studies to the lives and experiences of students?
13. Am I assisting students to work out a satisfactory compromise between the rigorous of abstract thinking and the human need for satisfying emotional loyalties?
14. Am I assisting students to adjust their thought processes and attitude to the changes in the social world about them?
15. Do I arouse students' interests in my subject and acquaint them with its cultural and vocational values?
16. Do I set up a provocative environment for the reconstruction of experience, utilising many school and community resources?
17. Do I use community resources to like the subject with life?
18. Do I seek professional growth continuously by such procedures as study, travel, meeting professional conference, etc.?

B. Attitude of the Social Studies Teacher Towards Students

1. Do I provide every student in my class, work so suited to his abilities and needs that he can succeed with reasonable effort?
2. Do I treat my students with reasonable courteous considerations?
3. Do I respect each individual's personality?
4. Do I have faith in the realisation of the best potentialities of each individual?

5. Do I keep my classroom atmosphere free from an intensely competitive atmosphere?
6. Do I stimulate students to discover and evaluate their own ability, strengths and weaknesses and to meet difficulty or criticism in a constructive way?
7. Do I try to understand my students rather than to judge them?
8. Do I watch the trend of the developing interest and attitude of my students?
9. Do I respect the right of every student to have confidential information about himself withheld except when its release is authorised in his or public interest?
10. Do I avoid disparaging remarks about child which might undermine his confidence?

C. Attitude of the Teacher towards Democratic Principles

1. Am I an example of democratic values?
2. Do I act as a democratic group leader?
3. Do I organise democratic groups which widen the area of common concern and encourage social leader?
4. Do I provide conditions by which social control will come out of the group situation?
5. Do I arrange learning experiences which are based on the interests, capacitites and needs of the children and which have continuity with life?
6. Do I provide conditions out of which arise opportunities for co-operatively solving a wide variety of problems and evaluating outcomes?
7. Do I share in formulating the purposes, policies and methods of the school?
8. Do I try become integrated into the community through active participation in the social life of the group?
9. Do I aid in the achievement of new cultural patterns which extend freedom?
10. Do I discuss controversial issues from an objective point of view thereby keeping the class free from partisan opinion?

D. Attitude of the Social Studies Teachers towards Parents and Colleagues, etc.

1. Do I provide parents with information that will serve the best interests of children?
2. Am I discreet with information received from parents?
3. Do I adhere to any reasonable pattern of behaviour accepted by the community for a professional person?
4. Do I refrain from discussing confidential and official information with unauthorised person?
5. Do I deal with other members of the profession in the same manner as I myself wish to be treated?
6. Do I speak constructively of other teachers?
7. Do I honestly report to responsible persons matters involving the welfare of the students, the school system and the profession?
8. Do I accept no compensation from producers of instructional material when my recommendations effect the local purchase or use of such teaching aids?
9. Do I recognise that everyone has some strength and weakness?
10. Do I keep quiet when I see fault in others?
11. Do I pick appropriate time and opportunity to ask for help or advise from others?
12. Do I expect everything to go my own way?

REVISION QUESTIONS

1. What are the various characteristics and qualities of an ideal social studies teacher, Discuss.
2. A teacher can 'foster the qualities of ideal citizenship' examine the statement and comment.
3. What should be the attitude of a social studies teacher?
4. Why is general and liberal education necessary for a social studies teacher?
5. Write short note on social studies teacher's relationship with his pupils and his colleagues.

13

Education for Democracy

13.1 INTRODUCTION

The word "Democracy" is derived from the Greek word "demos" which means people and "cratia" which means government or rule. Thus *democracy* means 'rule or government of the people.'

Aristotle defined democracy as *government by the many.*

According to Abraham Lincoln, "Democracy is a government of the people, by the people and for the people." Accordingly every citizen has a share in the government of the country.

According to Bryce, "Democracy is a form of government in which ruling power is largely vested not in any one individual or in a particular class or classes, but in the members of a community as a whole."

From all these definitions it appears that democracy is only a form of government but it is not correct. Democracy also means a social organisation wherein all members of community enjoy political and social equality, without any distinction of birth, caste, colour, creed or religion.

Democracy is also an economic ideal and in this sense it refers to a system of society wherein every member has equal economic opportunities.

Thus we find that it is not possible to define democracy in its entirety but we can say that in its principle it consists of the philosophy and practice of respect for the individual and willingness to give consideration to the needs, feelings, points of view and characteristics of all. It is a way of living and organisation of community that has unity in its political, social and economic aspects.

According to Wolff, "A democratic society, is a society of free, equal, active and intelligent citizens, each choosing his own way of life for himself and willing that others should choose theirs."

Truly speaking democracy is the catchword of present day society.

13.2 VALUES OF DEMOCRACY

Some of the important values of democracy are as follows:

1. Equality

Democracy is based on the principle of equality between man and man. In a democratic society all individuals are considered as equals irrespective of his capacities, contribution to society etc. In a democracy every individual is provided equal political, social and economic opportunities.

2. Respect for Individuality

In a democratic setup each individual member of the society is allowed a full scope for self-development and self-realisation and he is respected in social life as an individual irrespective of his vocation. Same importance is given to a sweeper or a labourer as is given to a doctor or an engineer.

3. Fellow Feeling and Co-operation

A democratic society is concerned with the welfare of the humanity and it provides no room to any artificial division of society on the basis of caste, creed, religion etc. It is based on humility and cooperation. Each individual is a co-worker and is entitled to share and respect the wishes of others. It is an interdependent society that is based on the principle of fellow-feeling, love and brotherhood.

4. Toleration

Since our aim in democratic society is to provide for individual development so we must be prepared to tolerate individual differences. The members of a truly democratic society are ever willing to tolerate all different types of differences in religion, caste, colour, wealth, thought and practice etc. This tolerance is possible if one never thinks that his way is the only right way and those who differ from him are all in wrong. Thus, the cardinal principles of democracy are a sense of give and take, toleration and compromise among citizens.

5. Change through Persuation

In a democratic setup changes are always recognised and welcomed. Such a society change with the development of new points of view, new technique and new possibilities for human life. A true democrat has a firm belief in dynamic life and not in a static one. He sees a progress in every change. He possesses a scientific attitude of life and tries to find out new truths. He believes in bringing about the desired change by persuation and not by force. The change in a democratic government can be easily brought about quite easily through peaceful and constitutional means. The conduct of a democratic society is always in conformity with the wishes of its citizens.

6. Self-education

Since democracy is a government by the people for their welfare so it teaches the individual to sacrifice his narrow, personal interests for the common good of all. The individual of a democratic society acquires certain moral values such as honesty, integrity, self-reliance, courage etc. For strengthening of democratic values the individual is expected to have a certain degree of intelligence, public spirit and discipline.

In the words of Woodrow Wilson, these virtues, "give a people self-possession, self-mastery, the habits of order and peace, the reverence for law which will not fail when they themselves become the makers of law and the steadiness and self-control of political maturity."

From the above discussion it becomes amply clear that democracy develops intellectual and spiritual qualities of man. It makes him interested in his country and infuses in him a sense of responsibility.

13.3 RELATIONSHIP BETWEEN DEMOCRACY AND EDUCATION

For the proper functioning of any democracy the basic requirement is that all the members of the community are provided education at least upto a certain minimum standard. In democracy education cannot be considered as a monopoly of only a few well-to-do or previleged people and it has to be considered as the birth right of all the members of a democratic society. Since in democracy each individual is equally important and he is expected to an intelligent use of his rights and to make his contribution to the welfare of the society so the democratic ideals must enter the life of an individual and it is possible only through his education. For imbibing democratic principles in the individual members patience and continuous educational efforts are needed. It is only by these that it is possible to create self-discipline and self-control among individuals or groups.

Just as democracy requires education, education also requires democracy because it is democracy that supplies the aims of education. The present day society aims at the production of democratic citizens. Thus education and democracy are functionally related to each other.

13.4 FUNCTION OF SCHOOLS IN A DEMOCRACY

The schools, in a democratic society, are expected to develop worthy interests in the child so that he is able to enrich his personality and improve his conduct. These worthy interests will make the child happy, well balanced and efficient citizen.

In the words of Ross, ''Schools ought to stress the duties and responsibilities of individual citizens. They ought to train their pupils in a spirit of cheerful, willing and effective service. They will teach citizenship directly and also through history. Every where there will be a spirit of team work, involving, a certain amount of self-derived; always the emphasis will be laid on the community. The true function of a school in a democracy, therefore, is to provide for the enrichment of the individual life for the child as he is now and to secure it for him when he grows up.''

By democratic education the child will not only learn about the successful operation of the democratic machineries but also the creation of democratic personalities. It has not yet been possible for us to develop democratic character in our country. The school is expected to play a frontal role and to act as the prime agent for society in this training.

13.5. AIMS OF DEMOCRATIC EDUCATION

The aims of democratic education in India as suggested by the Secondary Education Commission are as follows:

1. Developing Democratic Citizenship

The aim of education is to give a practical training of citizenship to the students. It should inculcate in young souls the democratic outlook. For our young democracy the teaching of social studies can help a lot to develop proper attitudes in young pupils, which can ultimately strengthen our democracy.

For strengthening of democracy it is desirable that an individual is able to distinguish between truth and falsehood and between fact and propaganda. Education should also inculcate in him the qualities of discipline, cooperation, social sensitiveness and tolerance. In a democracy the education must also aim at development of a sense of patriotism. Patriotism here does not only mean love and service of one's country but it also includes love and appreciation of the social, cultural and political advancement of the neighbouring countries and other countries of the world. The motto of a true patriot is "Live and Let Live."

2. Improvement of Vocational Efficiency

One of the important aims of education is to inculcate in our young souls a *sense of dignity of labour*. They should consider work as the very basis of all social progress. To inculcate the sense of dignity of labour in our students, craft has been allotted a prominent place. If the diversification of courses is allowed after say standard eight, it will enable the young pupils to select the vocation of their own taste and liking. It will be quite useful for attaining the aim of producing trained and efficient personnel to work out and carry out various schemes of industrial, technical and administrative advancement in our country.

3. Development of Personality

Development of personality is another important aim of education. With this aim in view an effort is made to develop creative energy among our students so as to enable them to appreciate their cultural heritage, to contribute to its development in later life and cultivate such interest to be pursued to their leisure.

In the words of Sir Percy Nunn, "Educational effort must be limited to securing for every one the conditions under which individuality is most completely developed-- that is enabling him to make his original contribution to the variegated whole of human characteristic as his nature permits; the form of contribution being left to the individual as something which each must, in living and by living, forge out for himself."

4. Education for Leadership

For a successful functioning of democracy all its citizens must be trained to discharge their responsibilities to the best of their ability and capacity. For this they should be given a training in discipline and leadership. The elementary school should provide training for disciplined work through craft whereas the university should provide training in leadership at the highest level, through multifarious activities.

K.G. Saiyidain summarises as "Education must be so oriented that it will develop the basic qualities of character which are necessary for the functioning of democratic life. These basic qualities are a passion for social justice, a quickening of social conscience, tolerance of intellectual and cultural differences, a systematic cultivation of critical intelligence, the development of love for work and a deep and true love for the country."

13.6 EDUCATION FOR DEMOCRACY THROUGH SOCIAL STUDIES

The effective teaching of democracy is quite difficult and is therefore a great challenge to any school and teacher. The Report of Secondary Education Commission in India recommends the inclusion of Social Studies as a core subject upto high school stage for meeting the challenge of effective teaching of democracy. It has been observed,

"Through this subject, the students should be able to acquire not only the knowledge but attitudes and values which are essential for group living and civic efficiency. It should endeavour to give the students not only a sense of national patriotism and an appreciation of national heritage, but also a keen and lively sense of world unity and world citizenship."

So the main burden to impart education for democracy has to be borne by the Social Studies teacher. He can carry out this job by undertaking the following programmes.

1. Creating Learning Situations

A good Social Studies can create such natural situations, for his pupils, which are conducive to good cooperative work and healthy human relationship. These situations help the child to learn by doing and experiencing in group life. Each one in the group is quite clear about his relationship and responsibility to the group. The group also understands its responsibility to the individuals. With these situations a student gets quite familiar with techniques of democratic procedure and deep appreciation of liberty, enjoyed by citizens of a nation.

2. Providing Definite Knowledge and Concepts

For providing the knowledge about certain concepts the subject-matter from civics and political science has to be included in the curriculum of Social Studies. With the help of this subject-matter that pertains to democracy as a form of government, as a social, economical and ethical idea and as a way of life, the teacher will be able to throw light on the rights and duties of citizens. Teacher can also suggest reading material, deliver lectures, undertake other activities for giving a direct knowledge and concepts related to democracy.

3. Providing Practical Experiences in Democratic Procedures

Activities of various types form an integral part of a course in Social Studies. Some of the teaching methods are based on such activities. These activities provide practical experience in electing, holding office, participating in community work, accepting group responsibility, assuming and discharging individual responsibility, acceding to the will of the group and taking decisions on controversial issues through discussion and mutual understanding. All this is an effective training for democracy.

4. Developing Desirable Skills and Attitudes

One of the aims of education is to develop right attitudes and skills as these are significant factors of behaviour. Attitudes are based on appreciation of things which are worthwhile in life. In social studies an effort is made to develop in students the desirable attitudes of co-operation, self-control, patience, sympathy, obedience, understanding and appreciation of differences, toleration, honesty and truthfulness etc.

The desirable skills which are expected to be developed by teaching of social studies are drawing and preparing maps, charts, graphs, models, pictures, cartoons, time lines etc.

13.7. CONCLUSION

To conclude it must be emphasised that to provide democratic education is a joint responsibility of school, home and society. Thus all out efforts be made to organise all relationships of an individual in accordance with democratic values. It has also been remarked, that, "Democracy is easy and fluid bending to the will of the people, changing with times and adjusting itself to meet new situations. Under it the supreme ideal is not the good of the state, the nation or the race but the good of the common people."

REVISION QUESTIONS

1. List some important values of democracy and discuss them in brief.
2. What is the relationship between education and democracy? Explain.
3. Give in brief the aims of education for democracy.
4. How can you impart the education for democracy by teaching of Social Studies.
5. Discuss the role of school in a democracy.
6. Write an essay on education for democracy.

14

Education for Citizenship

14.1 INTRODUCTION

The present age is an age of democracy and for successful functioning of democracy, we need an educational system which provides not only for needs of an individual but also for the needs of society. The educational system is expected to produce well-informed citizens who are familiar with public problems and who can keenly observe the activities of their elected representatives. They must also be conscious of their rights and obligations.

The educational programme is expected to produce, "citizens of the future who will take a common interest and active part in good government as well as exercise a high and fearless morality in their social relationship."[1]

The educational programme must be adjusted in accordance with the social and economic changes brought in by advances in science and technology, development in the means of transport and communication etc.

To understand the role of education in training of good citizenship one should be very clear in his mind about the concept of citizenship, rights and duties of good citizens, etc.

14.2 CITIZENSHIP

Ordinarily "citizen" means a resident of a city. The origin of this term can be traced back to ancient Greece which had many a city-states. The inhabitants of these states were known as "citizens" because these states consisted only of single cities, with a very small

1. Binning and Binning, *Teaching Social Studies in Secondary School*, p. 316.

territory and population. The citizenship even in such a small territory was a privilege of the selected few; women, manual workers and slaves were not given citizenship rights. In the direct administration of their state only a few actual citizens participated.

The use of the term "citizenship" has undergone a drastic change since those days and nowadays the term refers to all those members of the population of a state who enjoy all political and civil rights under the protection of the state in return of their loyalty to the state. The state protects the citizen's life, property, liberty etc. The state also provides to its citizens every opportunity for development of his personality and for leading a happy and useful life. The citizenship in modern times is "a legal relationship which binds an individual to the state of which he is a member."

Presently the citizenship is considered as the birth right of those persons who belong to a state. The states of today are not confined to single cities. They have a large population, an extensive territory, both urban and rural.

Importance of Citizenship

Citizenship demands from an individual to consider himself to be a part of the community and must be prepared to share its burdens and responsibilities. Ideally speaking he always puts the interest of the community before his personal interests and is always willing to sacrifice his own interests, wishes, conveniences, energy etc., for the sake of his community. It simply means that he is ready to sacrifice his personal interests for the sake of his family, his family interests for the sake of his community, his community interest for the sake of his nation and even the interest of the nation for the sake of larger humanity.

The above discussion makes it quite clear that citizenship is much more than paying taxes or performing one's duty as a member of a community or a nation. Its spirit, i.e., spirit of citizenship flows like blood in the veins of a nation.

World Citizenship

International understanding is equated with *world citizenship.* It implies mutual understanding, faith and respect among the various nations or countries of the world. In this age of science and technology no country can remain aloof and unconcerned from other countries because whatever is happening in one country, inevitably has its repercussions felt in other countries as well. This has necessitated mutually good and cordial relation amongst the countries of the world, which is termed international understanding or world citizenship.

Thus the citizenship is not confined to one particular state or nation but to the whole world community because the world is now-a-days one single unit -- one federation of all the nations.

Democracy and world citizenship are very closely connected with each other. In the definition of world citizenship the word "democracy" is of particular significance. Democracy is a **must** in world citizenship and training for civic responsibility in a democracy is a phase of world citizenship. Here it must be made clear that there is no clash between national citizenship and world citizenship. World citizenship is only an extended form of national citizenship.

Brimble and May, clarifying the point have observed in their book, *Social Studies and World Citizenship*, "If we consider the attributes of a good citizen in any community -- one who conducts his affairs with due regard for the welfare of the community of which he is a member and who is active and intelligent in his co-operation with his fellow members for the common good."

14.3 RIGHTS AND DUTIES OF A CITIZEN

The state protects the rights of a citizen and gives him freedom to act in any way for his fullest development in all respects such as physical, moral, intellectual etc. However, these rights have corresponding duties. These days we observe that every one lays emphasis on his rights and pays no need to his duties. However, one should never forget that if the rights imply a man's claim on society, duties indicate what he owes to society. It means that one owes to society as much as he claims from it.

The rights and duties of a citizen may differ from state to state but there are certain fundamental rights and duties which are almost universal. These fundamental rights include

(i) Right to life.

(ii) Right to liberty

(iii) Right to property

(iv) Right to work

(v) Right to education

(vi) Freedom of the press

(vii) Freedom of worship and

(viii) Freedom of association

The fundamental rights also include

(i) Right to vote

(ii) Right to election of legislature

(iii) Right to hold public office

(iv) Right to resist.

The list of duties of a citizen include

(i) Loyalty to the state

(ii) Obedience to law

(iii) Payment of taxes

(iv) Assistance in the administration of the state.

14.4 NEED FOR THE EDUCATION FOR CITIZENSHIP

Our common observation that individuals are more conscious of their rights and care a little for their duties compels us to remind them of their responsibilities and duties. For this we have to impart education for citizenship to every citizen/future citizen. The education for citizenship must be imparted to promote the cause of liberty and democracy.

Aldous Huxley has remarked, "If your goal is liberty and democracy, you must teach people, the arts of being free and governing themselves."

Citizens are to be trained and such a training should inculcate in them a sense of social responsibilities. To achieve this social function of education a special environment has to be created by the schools. The school is expected to serve as a living society for the rising generation of future citizens.

14.5 CITIZENSHIP EDUCATION THROUGH SOCIAL STUDIES

One of the main aims of social studies teaching in schools is the development of democratic citizenship among the younger generation. To-day when we talk of international understanding on which the very survival of humanity depends, we aim at securing an everlasting peace amongst the nations of the world. This aim of education can be achieved through the subject of social studies. In the study of social studies the child realises the interdependence of man and the desirability of reciprocal good-will.

The education in citizenship can be imparted through social studies as follows:

1. By Giving Definite Knowledge of Civic Competence

Teaching of social studies aims at generating political consciousness in the students. It should make them socially efficient. They should be well aware of the social and political problems of the country and should try to take active part in them. It is the students of today on whom depends the future of the country. Social efficiency requires the young students to have the qualities of sympathy, cooperation, patriotism etc. Such qualities can be developed in pupils only by teaching of social studies in a scientific manner. Factual knowledge quickens imagination and helps in building up individual interests. Definite knowledge about the past and present societies, develop a civic and historical background which enables young men and women to deal with new issues as they arise and think clearly about goals for the future. The teaching of social studies also makes an individual alert to his duties.

2. By Developing Primary Group Values

For a training in citizenship, one of the important steps is to develop primary group values. School can be considered as a miniature society and in it the students can be given basic training for citizenship. Students when asked to learn in groups and committees learn the lessons of honesty, obedience to law, cooperation, tolerance, self-control, self-sacrifice etc. Teacher should see that each individual is given a chance to have a status in a group and this status be recognised and respected by others. It will be quite helpful to an individual to learn that he has certain duties as also certain rights. It will also make him understand that others also have certain rights. In this way he will learn about the rights and duties of a citizen.

3. By Creating and Presenting Real Life Situations in Schools

The factual knowledge of the child must be supplemented by providing him actual democratic living in school. For this the students be put in actual life situations which can effectively put their civic sense to test. When students are put in actual life situations, they assume responsibility, show proper respect for rights of others, work in cooperation, play the role of leaders and followers, share and contribute express opinions fearlessly and settle differences by mutual understanding. It is the most effective and practical method to impart education in citizenship.

4. By Extending Civic Activities into the Community

If we can extend the pupil's activities into local community at work, it can provide a direct experience, to the child, in civic affairs. The pupils be encouraged to visit zoos, museums, art-galleries, courts, places of historical importance, places of geographical importance, places of economic importance, municipal halls, etc. They may be asked to see the election booths at the time of panchayat election, municipal elections or elections to assemblies and parliament. A tour be organised to the parliament house when parliament is in session. All these activities will help the pupils to understand how different groups of people in the community are engaged in the welfare of the community as a whole and what is their own duty in this direction.

5. By Developing Desirable Attitudes and Skills through Progressive Methods of Teaching

To develop desirable patterns of conduct is the basic aim of citizenship education. To attain this aim we have to develop in the pupils right attitudes and skills which are significant factors of behaviour. It is based on the appreciation of worthwhile things. Attitudes also depend on intellectual and emotional factors. Thus, the desirable attitudes are directly related to emotional well-being and balance. In a good citizen we expect attitudes such as sympathy, fellow feeling, patience, self-control, self-respect, tolerance, cooperation, obedience etc., which are consistent with principles and ideals of a democratic society. Skills of critical thinking and problem solving are also desirable in the citizens of a democratic set up. For development of these desirable attitudes and skill the training is imparted by adopting teaching of social studies through progressive methods such as the Project method, the problem method, the source method etc. All these methods put more emphasis on cooperative work and group activities. They develop group consciousness and the feeling of individual responsibilities towards the group.

14.6 ROLE OF THE TEACHER

In the programme of citizenship education the teacher is expected to play a significant role. To play his role effectively teacher should make a careful study of individual children, take a broad view of his teaching duties, make learning interesting, realistic and worth while. He should be concerned with the development of desirable attitudes and skills alongwith intellectual development. It is also his function to observe that each individual child applies the understanding, attitudes and skills of good citizenship in his daily life in and outside the class-room. To achieve all this the teacher must chalk out an instructional programme in such a way that it may put more stress on such features which are conducive to making up a democratic citizenship. He should always remember that the proof of good learning is found in good living.

REVISION QUESTIONS

1. Discuss in brief the rights and duties of a good citizen.
2. Why is social studies, as a school subject, considered so important for training of citizenship.
3. What do you understand by the term "citizenship?" What is its importance in present day world?
4. Bring about clearly the need of education for citizenship. Suggest a few practical measures to make such an education effective.
5. To what extent is it the duty of the school to provide efficient training in citizenship.

15

Education for International Understanding

15.1 INTRODUCTION

The term "International understanding" implies mutual understanding, faith and respect among various nations of the world. With the development of the supersonic means of transportation and communication, all the countries of the world have come closer to each other. Consequently no country can remain aloof and unconcerned from other countries because whatever is happening in one country, inevitably has its repercussions felt in other countries as well. This has necessitated mutually good and cordial relations amongst the countries of the world, which is termed as 'international understanding'.

15.2 VARIOUS DEFINITIONS OF INTERNATIONAL UNDERSTANDING

Some of the definitions of international understanding are as follows:

Oliver Goldsmith defines it "International understanding or Internationalism is a feeling that the individual is not only a member of his state, but a member of the world."

In the opinion of Walter H.C. Lewis, "International Understanding is the ability to observe critically and objectively, and apprise the conduct of man every where to each other, irrespective of the nationality or culture to which they may belong. To do this one must be able to detach oneself from one's own particular culture and national prejudices and to observe means of all nationalities, cultures and races as equally important varieties of human beings inhabiting this earth."

Dr. Atmanand Mishra opines "International understanding refers to friendship and harmony amongst different nations of the world and also includes cooperation amongst them -- each one maintaining its identity and sovereignty as usual."

In the words of Dr. Radhakrishnan, "The world, once divided by oceans and continents, is united physically today, but there are still suspicions and misunderstandings. It is essential for us not to live apart but to live together, understanding one another's fears and anxieties, aspirations and thoughts, that is what we are expected to do. We must not claim a racial extermination, enslavement or segregation, but work for racial harmony. We may be Germans, we may be Americans, we may be Russians, but we are essentially human beings. Let us not overlook that fundamental fact. Let us learn to live in world community." This is the idea of internationalism or international understanding.

International understanding in brief may thus be defined as "Informed consciousness of the place of one's own that it can make to world society, whose survival depends upon maintenance of peace and relief from war."

15.3 IMPORTANCE OF INTERNATIONAL UNDERSTANDING IN THE PRESENT WORLD

In the present age of science and technology international understanding is of vital importance as the very survival of humanity depends upon international understanding. The concept of international understanding aims at securing everlasting peace amongst the nations of the world which has become the most significant need of present world.

At present the necessity of establishing lasting peace among the nations is felt by all of us. It has been made clear, by the two world wars that we are sitting on the top of a volcano and if the leaders of the world fail to inculcate an attitude of peaceful coexistence, the consequences will be far deadlier than those even known in the history of mankind. This makes it absolutely imperative to bring about international understanding amongst the nations of the world. The problem of international understanding is becoming increasingly important because with the modern scientific weapons for destruction, another war may mean the end of present civilisation and humanity. If we wish to create peace and prosperity in our country, we must create good living conditions all over the world. It necessitates that we inculcate the idea of internationalism in minds of men. In the words of Pandit Jawaharlal Nehru, "Isolation means backwardness and decay. The world has changed and old barriers are breaking down; life becomes more international, we have to play our part in this coming internationalism."

Need of International Understanding

International understanding is needed because of the following reasons:

(i) To prevent world wars

(ii) To maintain one's sovereignty

(iii) To strengthen democratic principles

(iv) To develop backward nations

(v) To develop contacts with other countries

(vi) To promote human welfare.

After the removal of geographical barriers among the nations of the world, there is a strong desire among them to have greater collaboration and cooperation with one another. The urgency of this collaboration and cooperation has greatly increased on account of the economic factors. All the countries of the world are economically interdependent upon each other. No country is economically self-sufficient. Now there is an increasing realisation among all the nations of the world that the world shall fall or stand together. It makes clear the importance of international understanding.

15.4 NEED FOR TEACHING WORLD UNDERSTANDING IN SCHOOLS

The idea of international understanding has come to fore after the defeat of forces of narrow and aggressive nationalism at the hands of democracy in the Second World War which proved to be the most destructive war. It was thus felt that to save the world from the impending disaster, all the nations must commit themselves unequivocally to a world order wherein no nation is allowed to repudiate its professions of peace. Following factors are responsible for such a realisation.

1. Fear and Insecurity

The experiences of Second World War have made people, all over the world, fearful of the consequences of another international conflict. This fear arises due to the likelihood of untold sufferings and immeasurable destruction and devastation which an atomic war may bring in its make. A small energy falling in undesirable hands may bring about the end of humanity. It was precisely to avoid such an eventuality that the U.N.O. was formed. The chief aim of United Nations Organisation (U.N.O.) is "to save succeeding generations from the scourge of war, which twice in our life time has brought untold sorrow to mankind." This is possible only if nations seek to solve their differences and disputes through peaceful means and mutual understanding.

2. Economic Reasons

In the present age we find that no nation is economically self-sufficient and all nations are interdependent for resources and markets. In the past economic problem was solved through colonial expansion. Big powers established their colonies in the backward areas of the world. These colonies served as suppliers of raw materials at quite cheap rates and provided a ready market for the finished goods. Because of the political awakening during twentieth century the colonies and backward areas all over the world became independent nations. They could no more be exploited for 'economic gains' by the so-called "Imperial powers." Advances in science also brought the nations together by providing very fast means of transportation and communication. It resulted in expansion of markets and the economic activities of any nation cannot remain aloof. This economic inter-relationship and prosperity demands a clear understanding of the markets and peoples who constitute these markets. It clearly points to the need and importance of educating people for international understanding.

3. Humanitarian Reasons

In the present day society the need of international understanding is felt even on humanitarian grounds. The human nature is same every where as has been proved by recent researches in anthropology, sociology and psychology. It has also been proved beyond doubt that cooperation and non-aggression is the real nature of man. Aggression was accepted as a universal characteristic of society because of a defective social organisation. We have been compelled, by this realisation, to replace competetive society by a cooperative society.

A lasting peace is not possible if one part of the world is free and another part is slave, if one part is highly advanced and the other is utterly backward, if one part is economically prosperous and the other is so poor that in it even bare necessities of life are not available.

It has now been recognised that there are certain fundamental rights to which every one is entitled, irrespective of his caste, creed, colour, religion or nationality etc. Some of these are personal liberty, freedom, dignity, respect and good standard of social and economic life. If we wish to survive we must learn to live together and must not persist in our struggle for political power and economic superiority.

Education can play an important role in this direction. To transform the society from individualistic to the cooperative and planned society, education must rebuild the habits and attitudes of the people. Education must become the chief instrument for the realization of goals, accepted jointly by all nations of the world. It is only education and education alone that can stimulate intelligent curiosity, provide right moral values and create a profound sense of unity among human beings. A truly educated nation is one which is not dominated by group prejudices, party factions, intolerance, selfishness, injustice, individualism and exploitation. It is for these objectives that educational system of all nations be reoriented on these lines. The world is in transition from *nationalism* to *international civilisation*. Education can expedite this process and school is an important agency for this purpose.

15.5 IMPORTANT PRINCIPLES ON WHICH EDUCATION FOR INTERNATIONAL UNDERSTANDING IS TO BE BASED

Education for international understanding should be based on the following principles:

1. Developing the Capacity of Independent Thinking

The first and the foremost principle on which education for international understanding should be based is the developing and cultivating the power and capacity of independent thinking in our young men and women, so that they may be able to understand that above all, the world needs peace today. Peace leads to progress and happiness while war leads to destruction and misery. With their capacity for independent thinking, the youth will not be led by false propaganda. They will refuse to be misled by war mongers. They will be able to judge the statements of others before accepting them. They will be able to distinguish between truth and propaganda. They will also understand the importance of living in peace.

2. Developing Tolerance and Mutual Cooperation

"Live and let live" should be the guiding principle of all the nations of the world. If it can be accomplished then mistrust and suspicion will vanish and it will help to avoid war. The cause of international frictions is lack of mutual understanding. To avoid war we must lay more stress on ideas of cooperation and tolerance in our educational programme.

3. Interdependence of Mankind

Education of international understanding should stress the idea of interdependence of nations. It must be made clear to the child that no nation these days can live by itself. Each nation has to depend on other nations of the world for one thing or the other. No country in modern world can afford to live in isolation. Each nation may be a separate political entity but they are economically knit together. The needs of all nations can be better satisfied through international understanding and cooperation.

4. Redefining Patriotism

The term "patriotism" should not be conceived in its narrow sense because such a concept is very dangerous for international peace. In its narrow sense, patriotism means exalting one's own country above all others and ignoring the achievements of other countries. The slogan "My country -- right or wrong" stands no where in the present day society. True patriotism means loyalty to one's own country provided this loyalty does not clash in any way with the interests of the other countries. The love of one's country should not stand in the way of wider loyalty to humanity. Therefore, the word patriotism should be redefined and reinterpreted so that it is wide enough and consistent with internationalism. True patriotism is wider loyalty to humanity.

5. Elimination of Fear

Fear is the basis of mutual suspicion of nations which leads to race for armament. Being afraid and suspicious of one another the nations prepare themselves for war. Fear can be removed through proper training and education by stressing the principle of "Live and let live". In the words of Bertrand Russel, "the universal apprehension is itself a potent cause of war." Hence, fear should be eliminated from individual and national life.

6. Practical Use of Knowledge

Only theoretical knowledge is not sufficient. We have to train our young men and women to apply their theoretical knowledge in their daily life. For education to become successful the fact must be converted into a faculty, information should ripen to wisdom and desirable behaviour. By the application of knowledge the young citizens are able to understand that the principle of human relationship which hold good in the internal working of their country also holds good in international sphere. The knowledge of one's religion is not sufficient, one should try to live according to the teachings of his religion but he must also show due regards to the religious beliefs of others. Such actions can unite us in the bonds of spiritual unity of mankind.

7. Belief in Universal Freedom

We have left behind the time of imperialism, colonialism and capitalism. The present day society does not permit any nation to subjugate other nations, politically or economically. We are living in an age of democracy and it provides maximum individual freedom consistent with general welfare. These days we consider freedom as the birth right of every individual. However, freedom must not be considered as a licence nor simply removal of restraints. Freedom is the product of discipline. In a democracy freedom is restricted both by the obligation of one citizen to the other as also by the capacities of an individual to use his freedom for self-development and common good. Freedom is thus a goal to be reached after vigorous training in responsible activity and such a training can best be provided in the school through a planned system of education.

8. Inculcate Corporate Responsibility

In the opinion of Prof. K.G. Saiyidain, education for international understanding should be based on the principle of corporate responsibility. We must teach our children to believe that they are citizens of the world which is one and indivisible. In this world if we have anything bad or ugly, we all are equally responsible for it. We all must work in unison for the achievement of common aims. Good men and good citizens are those who freely accept responsibilities. Civilization is only an impulse towards ordering our lives on the basis of discussion, understanding and coexistence. Let our education make us realise that we all are brethren and as such we must help another in times of difficulty and distress. Education will provide necessary training in this behalf.

9. Emphasis on Correct Values

Education for international understanding should be based on the principle of emphasizing correct values. Democratic values, group responsibility, tolerance, cooperation, mutual understanding etc. should be stressed and impressed upon the students. It should be impressed upon pupils that they are world citizens and that they belong to entire world. Thus we should create faith for humanity in their minds. Humanity is the true religion of human beings, while all the great religions are only its different forms. We must impress upon our students that man is the most beautiful creation of the universe and basically we like goodness and peace. The end of education should therefore be the cultivation of intellectual and spiritual values, bringing to a maximum development, the moral potentialities of man.

Principles as Recommended by UNESCO

According to the UNESCO report, it is imperative to:

(i) make it clear that unless steps are taken to educate mankind for the world community, it will be impossible to create an international society conceived in the spirit of the charater of United Nations;

(ii) make clear that States, whatever their differences of creeds and ways of life, have both a duty to cooperate in international organisations and interest in doing so;

(iii) make clear that civilization results from the cultivation of many nations and that all nations depend very much on each other;

(iv) make clear the underlying reasons which account for the changing ways of life of different peoples, their past and present, their traditions, their characteristics, their problems and the ways in which they have been resolved;

(v) make clear the engagements freely entered into by the member states of international organisations have force only insofar as they are actively and effectively supported by those peoples;

(vi) arouse in minds, particularly of young people, a sense of responsibility to this world community and to peace.

(vii) encourage the development of healthy social attitudes in children so as to lay the foundations of international understanding and cooperation.

15.6. MEANS OF IMPARTING EDUCATION FOR INTERNATIONAL UNDERSTANDING

Education is a powerful force in developing internationalism. In the words of Bertrand Russel, education may not bring internationalism from political point of view but education is the only agency through which it is possible to develop the feeling of internationalism. Therefore, education should be so organised and formulated that it may promote international understanding. The following are some of the ways and means of organising education for promoting the feelings and thoughts of internationalism.

1. Reorienting Curriculum and Text-books

For promoting the feeling of internationalism, the first step should be the reorientation of the educational curriculum and the text-books. It is through the right type of curriculum and text-books that the children's mind can be reoriented in the direction of peace and international understanding. Hence while redesigning the curriculum, the aim of developing international understanding among students must be kept in view. The redesigned curriculum should enable the students to acquire the following knowledge:

(a) Knowledge of interdependence of different countries of the world.
(b) Knowledge of similarities of ideas and moral ideals propagated by different religions of the world.
(c) Knowledge of various cultures of the world.
(d) Knowledge of entire world, its countries and people, their ways of living and thinking.
(e) Knowledge of the struggle of mankind for the establishment of peace.

Thus all the school subjects like history, geography, civics, economics etc. should initiate the students into wider world of which they are the members. The children of today are the citizens of tomorrow, writes C.D. Deshmukh, in his book "Education for International Understanding". It is in their minds that must take root ideas, leading to the realization of the common heritage of man, an understanding and appreciation of differences among peoples, a recognition of the basic human dignity which must be respected and safeguarded, an awareness of the interdependence of nations and the consequent need of international understanding."

Social Studies has been introduced as a core subject upto high school stage with the definite aim of creating a realization of interdependence of man and man and nation and nation as well as to promote international understanding and respect for humanity. This is a subject which aims at developing among children the individual and social virtues of initiative, self-reliance, faithfulness, righteousness, constructive thinking, critical judgement, justice, tolerance, cooperation and feeling for making them reliable associates and trusted neighbours. Social studies, therefore, is the most important subject for teaching world understanding and international coexistence. This aim can be best achieved by making international understanding as the core or central theme round which the entire subject-matter and activities of social studies should revolve. This is possible through the following means:

1. Definite Knowledge and Information

With the help of social studies teaching it is possible to make our students understand and appreciate the contributions made by different nations towards the cultural heritage of mankind. It is the culture of a nation that makes it what it is. It is the nation's values that determine what it will do and what it will become. Thus from our knowledge of culture it is possible to appreciate these values. It can also help us to understand their differences from our own. So we can say that cultural understanding is the basis of all other types of understanding.

The physical side of social studies also makes it clear to the students that world is the home of the man, where all human beings have to live and satisfy the same basic needs, though with different means, depending upon their physical environments. It should also tell them how modern man has learnt to control or be controlled by physical environments and how far he has been successful in adapting himself to various social situations.

The pupil's relationship to his social environment is emphasized by civics and political science side of social studies and the economic aspect from the economics side of social studies. Thus, definite knowledge of various environments that affect human life will promote understanding of all history and all human experiences as a process of change and development will definitely lead to world understanding and international peace and harmony.

2. Proper Co-curricular Activities

International understanding can also be promoted through various types of cocurricular activities. These activities should include the celebrations of birthdays of great men and women belonging to different countries and religions like Gautam Buddha, Lord Christ, Mohammad, Guru Nanak, Lord Krishna, Newton, Marcony, Edison, Lenin, Gandhi, Tagore etc. The celebration of international days like the UNO day, the human rights day, the world health day etc. These will provide occasions to pupils for studying the composition, significance and activities of the UNO and its other agencies with regards to maintenance of international peace and security. Lectures by foreign scholars may be arranged from time to time. The school should also keep the students informed of the latest developments in the world through newspapers, magazines, journals, lectures and discussions etc. Films and film strips about the physical features, human activities and culture of other countries may also be screened.

3. Cultural Exchanges

Schools should cooperate and actively participate in the programme of sending cultural missions, consisting of teachers, students, scholars, poets, artists and writers etc. to different countries of the world. Such cultural tours to other countries can be frequently arranged. We can also invite foreigners to visit our country. It will rectify wrong notions and will create sympathy and affection for the people of other countries. This will also broaden the mental outlook of the people and will help in establishing cultural ties among various nations.

In the words of Dr. C.D. Deshmukh, one important means of furthering international understanding is ''international exchange of persons, directed not only with a view to facilitating the transmission of knowledge, skills and experiences, but also to encourage free and frank discussion of differences in such a way as to minimize the area of misunderstanding and to maximise that of cooperation. The programme in this behalf should lay stress on living together and benefitting from direct contacts.'' Pen friendship should also be encouraged.

4. Role of the Teacher

The personality of the social studies teacher is of utmost importance in imparting education for international understanding. He must have a clear understanding of the ideas, men and affairs. He must have an international outlook and be a man of broad mind and vision. He should see that all the school activities and methods of teaching are deeply influenced by the spirit of internationalism. It is he who presents curriculum from international point of view. He should enlighten students about life in various countries. He should also stress the need of international cooperation for the progress and prosperity of humanity as a whole. It is he who exposes the conflict between narrow nationalism and a rational and responsible international order. It is the responsibility of the teacher to careate strength of will and determination among the younger generation to enable it to stand boldly and successfully against those who believe that war is the only means of resolving differences among nations.

A study of UNO and its specialised agencies in the social and cultural fields, and the work done by them for India and other developing countries should be specially stressed in the classes. Thus it will be seen that teachers can participate in this project.

In the words of Dr. K.L. Shrimali, "If education is to be the instrument of social change, teachers cannot remain content in an attitude of vacillation and uncertainty. They must not only take sides but give leadership to the democratic forces in the world -- in Africa and Asia -- which are struggling for the freedom of common man. They must harness these forces for bringing into existence greater human solidarity, peace. Educational profession will become effective instrument for the safeguarding of civilization only to the degree that teachers are courageous, purposeful and united. They will be successful in educating the younger generation for international understanding only to the extent that they realise their own responsibility towards the world community."

15.7 CONCLUSION

International understanding is the need of the day. Education is a strong and potent agency for promoting international understanding. It is rightly said, that international understanding will not emerge from the science laboratories where atom bombs and other deadlier weapons are manufactured, but from the schools and colleges where human energy is directed into useful channels. Hence the spirit of peaceful coexistence and international harmony should pervade the whole of school and college life and learning. The process of developing international understanding is rather slow and difficult, but effort is worth doing. Not only progress and prosperity but the very survival of mankind is dependent upon promoting internationalism and international understanding. In the words of Gandhiji, "This world is bound to be doomed unless the lessons of love, truth and non-violence could find their way into the home and the school and thereby, eventually into the social, political and economic organisations of the world. If we want to change the world, we cannot do so merely by trying to change the outer world; we must also change the world within the world of *man's mind and emotions*, where the seeds of violence and hatred or peace and love, are initially sown."

The same idea is expressed in the preamble of the constitution of UNESCO in these words, "Since wars begin in the minds of men, it is the minds of men that the defence of peace must be constructed."

REVISION QUESTIONS

1. Explain the concept of international understanding.
2. Briefly explain the importance of international understanding in the present world.
3. Why do we need teaching of international understanding in schools?
4. State the main principles on which teaching of international understanding may be based.
5. How is it possible to develop international understanding among students through the subject of social studies?
6. Give various principles recommended by UNESCO for international understanding.
7. Discuss various ways and means for imparting education for international understanding.
8. Discuss the importance of social studies teacher in developing an international outlook among his pupils.

16

Evaluation in Social Studies

16.1 INTRODUCTION

Once a teacher has a clear view of what she will teach and how she will teach it, she is concerned with knowing to what extent children learn from her lessons. This chapter will deal with specific procedures for evaluating the effectiveness of social studies teaching-learning.

Evaluation is a continuous process which is an integral part of teaching. It is not merely a test at the end of a social studies lesson or unit. Instead, evaluation goes on constantly during lessons and units and is clearly related to the teacher's goal and points of view on geography teaching.

Besides being a continuous experience, evaluation is cumulative. A cumulative social studies record should be kept for all children. If such a record is available then his social studies exposure can be quickly and easily seen.

The recent trends in learning and evaluation link them to behavioural objectives. According to behaviourist psychology learning is defined as a *charge in the behaviour of an individual that can be described in terms of observable and measurable performance*. The changes in behaviour are affected by providing experiences and through teaching.

The test efficiency of teaching, to judge the progress of students and to discover their achievements and evaluate the whole school system, we require some sort of measuring tools. These tools are *tests or examinations*. Tests are sessential to grade and rank pupils, however, if evaluation is used merely to indicate areas of social studies to which children have been exposed or for classifying and categorizing students, a great value is lost. The same loss occurs if evaluation is interpreted only as arriving at numerical or alphabetical ratings for report cards. In this way much of the positive use of evaluation as a means of teaching and learning could be destroyed.

Effective instructional planning and evaluation of students' performance have always stressed upon statement of instructional objectives so that they are of great help to the student. According to Muller, an instructionally usable objective must state the intended outcome in terms of the terminal behaviour of students. Terminal behaviour here stands for the behaviour of students after the classroom instructions and evaluation can be made if the learning outcomes are carefully specific. By coupling continuous evaluation with immediate application of what has been learned, the teacher can provide for:

(i) The stimulation of students who learn rapidly to greater growth towards goals by application of advanced works.
(ii) The identification of specific weakness and difficulties in functional understanding (concepts, principles, generalisations) and the needed reteaching of varied activities, skills or problem solving abilities, and
(iii) The clarification, modification or complete alternation of the goals as needed for the unit.

Evaluation teaching and learning are the three corners of the education system. *Evaluation* is connected with finding out how far students have learned as a consequence of teaching. There are two kinds of evaluation depending upon whether the comparison of student is made with some absolute performance standard or with other students of a given group. These are known as *criterion referenced evaluation* and *norm reference evaluation.*

16.2 MEANING OF EVALUATION

Evaluation is the inclusive concept. It indicates all kinds of means to ascertain the quality value and effectiveness of desired outcomes. It is a compound of objective evidence and subjective observations. It is the total and lineal estimate... It is a valuable and indispensable guide to the modification of policies and to further action. In other words, we can say that evaluation is the approval of pupils progress, in attaining the educational goals set by the school, class and himself. The chief purpose of evaluation is to guide and further the student's learning. Evaluation is thus a positive rather than a negative process.

Evaluation, in fact, according to its latest concept rests upon three pillars, viz.

(i) education objectives

(ii) learning experiences and behaviour changes, and

(iii) tools and techniques of evaluation.

These can be represented diagramatically by means of the following triangle:

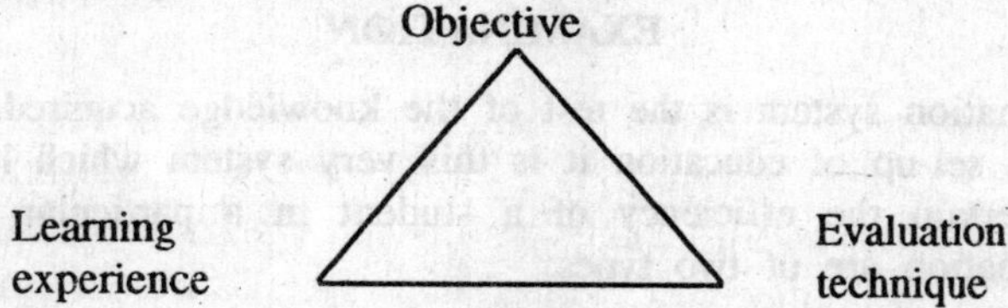

Objectives are central to both learning experiences and evaluation. Evaluation comes in at the planning stage when objectives are determined. Similarly learning experiences are also planned and organised in terms of objectives.

Evaluation must form an integral part of teaching because it is a continuous process, related to total learning situation. It indicates an inter-relationship among the society, the school, the body of knowledge, instruction and social behaviour. Evaluation is continuous and natural enterprise of all concerned.

Important Elements in Evaluation

Measurement and *appraisal* are the two principal elements in evaluation.

Measurement is the objective and exact part of evaluation which can be definitely ascertained and accurately measured with the help of a number of excellent tests.

Appraisal is the process of evaluating intangible qualities, characteristics, interests, attitudes and understandings. However, good tests in this area are rarely available. Moreover good techniques for measurement of attitudes, feelings, interests and values etc., are not available. Techniques of testing are reasonably effective in measuring individual persons attitudes, interests, feelings and values because these are specific to situations, which cannot be realistically produced by any test. So appraisal rests upon *observation* and *interpretation* and finally upon subjective opinion. Thus both measurement and appraisal are integral parts of evaluation. Neither of the two is more important than the other. Appraisal operates in those areas to which measurement cannot be applied. In fact, appraisal based upon records and concrete observations, has assumed some of the importance which was previously attached to measurement alone.

16.3 IMPORTANCE OF EVALUATION OR EXAMINATION

Examination system is the test of the knowledge acquired. In the present set-up of education it is this very system which helps us to ascertain the efficiency of a student in a particular subject. Examination are of two types:

(a) Written or theoretical, and

(b) Oral.

Written tests are 'essay type tests'. Probably it is the type of test which makes the students feel unhappy and nervous about their examination days. Various scholars have given various epithets to this type of examination. Some of these are given below:

1. A bane of educational system
2. A blood sucker
3. A necessary evil
4. An obstacle to learning
5. An enemy of true education etc., etc.

Examinations are conducted to measure the achievement. This measure of achievement is known as evaluation or *examination.* Unless we are able to have proper assessment and evaluation of the achievement. The achievement becomes meaningless. This process helps a person to improve his achievement. This is what shall be more clear from the following lines:

''Evaluation signifies a wider, more comprehensive and

continuous process of assessing student progress. It is integrated with the whole task of education and its purpose is to improve instruction and not merely to measure its achievement. In its highest sense evaluation brings out the factors that are inherent in student growth such as proper attitude and understanding."

There is some distinction between examination and evaluation. Examination is slightly less comprehensive while evaluation is more. In fact, evaluation is a new technical term. It connotes a comprehensive concept of measurement. J.W. Wrightstone has rightly remarked:

"Evaluation is a relatively new technical term introduced to designate a more comprehensive concept of measurement that is applied in conventional test and examinations. ... The emphasis in measurement is upon single aspects of subject-matter achievement or specific skills and abilities. ... The emphasis in evaluation is upon board personality changes and major objectives of an educational programme. This includes not only the subject-matter achievement but also attitudes, interests, ideals, ways of thinking, work habits and personal and social abilities."

In others words, it means that it is the evaluation examination that helps not only the improvement of the achievement but also improvement of different traits of personality.

16.4 PURPOSE OF EVALUATION

Evaluation fulfills the following purposes:

(i) It assesses the extent of learning by students and gives them the feed-back about their performance.

(ii) It gives feed-back to the teacher about the learning gaps of the students. It also provides the teacher a feed-back about the quality of his class-room instructions.

(iii) It provides the student an opportunity to show his worth.

(iv) It serves as a screening tool for selecting students for special purposes.

(v) To assess the success of educational system or the methods of teaching.

(vi) To provide educational, vocational guidance and counselling.

(vii) To examine the utility of the techniques and aids of teaching.

(viii) To find the aptitudes and inclinations of the students.

(ix) To encourage the process of learning.

(x) To bring about reforms in teaching and curriculum.

Our evaluation has another goal besides assisting the teacher in assessing and modifying her teaching procedures. This goal *self-evaluation* is not solely for the students. As teacher and students actively engage in all levels of a study such as initial planning, organisation and carrying out activities they can be guided in developing ability to evaluate themselves. Knowing the general and specific goals can aid the pupil in checking himself all along the way. This makes the learner an active participant in class-room activities. It also places some of the responsibility on him for learning and assessing what and how much he has learned. Self-guided evaluation stimulates healthy and realistic achievement goals. A logical first step in self-evaluations is setting up of realistic goals. These goals for civics teaching in elementary schools are:

(i) *Functional understandings* such as concepts, principles, generalizations, and the facts needed.

(ii) *Problem solving* skills such as defining problems, proposing hypotheses and techniques necessary for the solution of the problems, observational techniques, discussion and interpretations skills.

(iii) *Scientific attitudes, interests and appreciation* such as open mindedness and humanity.

The easiest are to evaluate is functional understanding because a rich variety of test are well-known and are widely used in elementary schools. Before we proceed to actual discussion of these tests let us consider the criterion of a good examination and prerequisites of a physical test.

16.5 SPECIAL OBJECTIVES OF EVALUATION IN SOCIAL STUDIES

The special objectives of evaluation in social studies are as follows:

(i) to help in measuring factual knowledge;

(ii) to help in diagnosing weakness;
(iii) to help in predicting future achievements;
(iv) to stimulate instructions;
(v) to meet criticism;
(vi) to test the development of skills and attitudes.

However, we find that most of the teachers are not serious about these objectives. They are either ignorant of them or are seldom interested in this important part of instructional process.

Most of the young social studies teachers are full of enthusiasm and zeal about their subject so long as they are under-training in training colleges. But soon after, they enter the teaching profession, they fall in the main stream and lose all their enthusiasm and zeal. In this way, the evaluation, which is very important part of educational process fails to serve its unique purpose. Teachers must remember that they will succeed in their aim to the extent to which they utilize and are guided by the result of evaluation.

16.6 CRITERIA OF A GOOD EXAMINATION

Though a variety of tests are available to test the functional understanding of the child but for true assessment of such aspects of growth as the elements of reflective things, scientific attitudes, resourcefulness, creativeness or such other objectives or interests we require more precise and accurate instruments of evaluation. According to most of the psychologists and educationalists the following are essential criteria of satisfactory evaluation.

1. *Validity*: Any good test should measure what it claims to measure.
2. *Reliability*: A good test is one that is reliable i.e., it gives same rating to a candidate even if he is examined by different examiners and even at different times.
3. *Objectivity*: A test can be considered objective if the scoring of the test is not affected in any way by the examiner's personal judgment. Thus the opinion, bias or judgment of the examiner can have no influence on the results of on objective test.
4. *Comprehensiveness*: By comprehensiveness of a test we mean that it covers the whole or nearly the whole course

content and the questions are uniformly distributed to cover the course content.

5. *Practicability:* A test is called practicable if it can be easily administered and is acceptable to average examiners. While preparing such a test, the time and cost of administration must be taken into consideration. The test should be usable and should serve a definite need in the situation in which it is used.
6. *Interpretability*: A test can be considered as interpretable if its score can be used and interpreted in terms of a common base having natural or accepted meaning.
7. *Easy to Administer*: A good test should be easy to administer so definite provision be made for collection and preparation of test material. It should give simple, clear and precise instructions.

Pre-requisites of a Good Test

There are certain pre-requisites for preparing a good test. These are as under:

Aspects	*Description*
1	2
Aims	— Acquisition of knowledge of various political concepts and skills.
	— Development of scientific attitude and interest.
	— Development of laboratory skills.
	— Highlighting the application of civics/politics in every day life.
	— Development of skills of information processing, observation, enquiry and design.
	— Acquisition of problem solving abilities.
Objectives	
(a) *Knowledge*	Recall and recognition of factual information such as
	(i) Definitions of various terms.
	(ii) Statement of laws, principles, rules, conventions etc.

1	2
	(iii) Description of construction and working of devices and instruments.
	(iv) Description of events, processes and phenomenon.
	(v) Recognising the parts of devices, instruments, appliances and apparatus.
	(vi) Identifying known physical phenomenon, events and occurrences.
(b) *Comprehension:*	Understanding facts, laws etc.
	(i) Comparing and contrasting various phenomenon.
	(ii) Locating error, limitations and defects.
	(iii) Illustrating scientific phenomenon.
	(iv) Reasoning events on the basis of certain principles and laws.
(c) *Applications:*	Using knowledge in new situations
	(i) Solving numerical problems.
	(ii) Making use of various laws in various situations and events.
	(iii) Relating various variables.
(d) *Skills:*	Using psycho-motor skills
	(i) Laying out an experimental set-up.
	(ii) Drawing diagrams, graphs, histograms, flow charts etc.
	(iii) Reading various measuring instruments.
(e) *Analysis:*	Breaking up information into parts of reach conclusions
	(i) Interpretation of observations.
	(ii) Drawing inferences from observations.
	(iii) Generalising conclusions.

1	2
(f) *Synthesis:*	Combining parts of information to grasp a concept (i) Designing an experiment (ii) Improvising an experiment, apparatus or device. (iii) Improving the accuracy of an instrument.

16.7 EVALUATING THE RESULTS OF SOCIAL STUDIES INSTRUCTIONS

An evaluation programme in Social Studies should include the following instruments:

1. *For Evaluating Knowledge, Information and Concepts*:
   (i) Oral tests
   (ii) Essay type tests
   (iii) Objective tests
   (iv) Testing the pupils' day to day work, in class.
2. *For Evaluating Skills, Interest and Values*:
   (i) Observation
   (ii) Conferences and interviews
   (iii) Anecdotal Records
   (iv) Diaries and Logs
   (v) Work samples
   (vi) Pupils' interest inventories
   (vii) Sociometry
   (viii) Objective standardized tests.
   (ix) Cumulative records.

1. Evaluation of Knowledge, Information and Concepts

(i) *Oral Tests:* This type of tests must form an integral part of the evaluation programme in social studies. However, we seldom make use of oral questioning in teaching-learning process and that is why that our students even at graduate and post-graduate levels cannot express themselves orally. To overcome this deficiency it is desirable that we use oral questioning in our teaching process to test the previous knowledge of the students. Such questions not only keep the student alert and attentive but also stimulate their mental activity. The teacher is also in a position to know whether his pupils are working seriously and regularly or otherwise. Oral questioning will serve its real purpose only if they are made an essential part of evaluation. For this the students have to be encouraged to express themselves orally as often and as nicely as possible. It will also help to develop in them the habit of public speaking which is an essential quality in a democracy. In any scheme of evaluation some marks should therefore be set aside for **oral** or **viva-voce** testing at the end of each term or whenever formal evaluation has to take place. Such questions should be put on the topics, covered by the students in the class, and they should be encouraged to answer those questions orally, within the time limit, already made known to them.

(ii) *Essay Type Tests:* This type of tests are designed to test pupils' knowledge of a particular subject as expressed in a limited number of questions of the discussion type. In case of Social Studies such tests occupy an important position. It is easy to prepare and administer such a type of test. Students are provided with opportunities to express themselves as fully as possible.

They can test a wide range of abilities including critical thinking, interpretation, reasoning power and judgement.

In it we can cover a wide range of subject of matter. To make these tests more objective questions on the construction of maps graphs, charts, time lives etc. should be set as important parts of evaluation through essay type tests.

It measures only the factual knowledge retained by the pupils. It is based on the power of memorisation and cramming and so it deprived the pupil of varied abilities. Attitude, emotions, interests have no place in such a type of examination programme.

The new idea of evaluation is more comprehensive and it includes the testing of both tangible and intengible qualities. It is related to total learning situation. It is meaningful process, utilising many resources as they apply to the objective of a democratic and forward looking structure. It takes into consideration the growth of a child as a whole individual and his total environment.

In evaluation one should know where the pupils were at the beginning of the teaching learning process, get a record of changes brought in them and judge how good those changes are in relation to previously established objectives. Evaluation is thus objective as well as subjective. It is a continuous and developing process which must form an essential part of a social studies programme. It must be made part of each problem and each unit of work in Social Studies and should relate to the objective of that unit or problem.

Traditional Types of Test or Traditional Type of Examination

It consists of only one form of questions and that is essay type questions.

Defects of Traditional Type of Tests or Examinations

At present new types of test are taking the place of traditional or essay type of tests. This trend is gaining importance because traditional type of examinations suffer from following defects:

(a) Defects from the Point of View of Students

(i) The essay type tests are less objective and so they lack validity. This type of test can reveal child's cramming capacity only.

(ii) These tests lack reliability. A student is compelled to have a selective reading. He depends more on guess papers and so there is an element of chance.

(iii) It keeps the students busy and full of nervous tension. The study does not spread over the whole year and is limited to a short period just before the examinations. Thus a habit of irregular study is developed in the student.

(b) Defects of Essay Type Examination from the Point of View of the Teacher

(i) The teacher covers only a limited and important portion of course because his aim is to see that maximum number of his students pass the examination.

(ii) The teaching programme of the teacher is wholly examination oriented and the basic principle of teaching his students are given least consideration.

(iii) The teacher is compelled to encourage his students to cramming which is not a psychological method of teaching.

(iv) Since a teacher is judge by the results of his students so every thing becomes subservient to the examinations.

(v) To show good results sometimes the teacher devotes a good deal of his time to indulge in guess work which affects his teaching.

(c) Defects from the Point of View of Achievement

(i) Essay type tests are not comprehensive and some students may get good marks only because the questions have been set from the portion prepared by them.

(ii) These tests are not objective and score of a student depends on various factors such as examiner's mood and whims etc.

(iii) This type of tests are not useful from the point of view of improvement. They fail to throw light on the defects of teaching-learning process or the defects of the curriculum.

From the above it can be concluded that essay type examination is not a correct method of evaluation in social studies. The improvement in system of evaluation is possible if following suggestions are given due consideration.

(a) Improvement in Essay Type Examination

In essay type examination an improvement is possible if we set shorter questions spread over the whole course. The language of question should be clear and precise, clear cut directions be given for scoring.

3. Objective Type Tests

The objective type tests form the latest technique in testing. They consist of the following type of tests:

1. Recall type of test.
2. Alternate response type of test.

3. Multiple choice type of test.
4. Matching type of test.
5. The completion type of test.
6. Classification type of test.

In addition to essay type tests, some objective type tests may also be used for evaluation. The objective type tests can be of the following types:

(a) True-false type.

(b) Completion type

(c) Multiple choice type.

(d) Matching type.

(e) Short answer type.

Objective type tests have the following merits:

(i) The objective tests have little or no scope of subjectivity. The score does not depend on Examiner's mood or whims.

(ii) These tests are more reliable. The score does not depend on expression, speed, style etc.

(iii) These are comprehensive. This requires from the students, thorough study of the syllabus.

(iv) There is no chance element in this type of test.

(v) These are easy to administer and easy to score.

(vi) These are economical in respect of time.

However, they also suffer from certain drawbacks. Some of these are as under:

(i) The objective type tests fail to test the organising ability of the students.

(ii) These tests fail to develop thinking and reasoning powers of the students which is one of the main aims of teaching social studies.

(iii) These tests put more emphasis on factual knowledge and very little importance is given to processes, methods or originality of thought.

(iv) These tests encourage guess work.

(v) These tests are not diagnostic. Because they do not show the defects in the teaching-learning process.

(vi) These tests may pose some administrative difficulties as there may be indiscipline in the students. They may use unfair means, wishper answers or make some gestures.

(vii) It needs a lot of time and labour for preparing such a test.

Different Types of Objective Tests

We have already seen the various types of objective tests. Let-us now describe each of them in some detail.

1. Recognition Type of Test

Through this method, an attempt is made to assess the power of recognition of the student. In this method the student has to find out the correct answer out of several answers given. There are several sub-forms of this type of tests. They are given below:

(a) Alternate response type or true/false test.

(b) Multiple choice test.

(c) Matching type test.

(d) Classification type tests.

(a) Alternate response type or true/false test: In this type of test, the answer is limited to the possibilities of true and false. Two alternatives are given and the examine has to choose one. Sometimes the signs of '√' and 'X' are also required to be used.

Example of the response type or true/false test:

Note: Given below are certain statements. Put the letter 'T' against the statements that are true and 'F' against the statements that are false:

1. Pakistan invaded India in 1965.
2. Dr. V.V. Giri is the Prime Minister of India.
3. The Prime Minister of India is elected by the people directly.
4. Mr. C.B. Gupta is the Chief Minister of Uttar Pradesh.

(b) Multiple choice type test: In this type of test, several answers are given to a particular question. The student is asked to find out the correct answer.

Example

Note: Given below are several answers to a particular question. Put the sign '✔' against the correct answer.

1. India secured freedom on January 26, 1948/August 15, 1947/ January 26, 1950.
2. Mrs. Vijai Laxmi Pandit/Mrs. Sucheta Kripalani/Mrs. Indira Gandhi/Mrs. Tarkeshwari Sinha/Mr. P.V. Narasimha Rao is the Prime Minister of India.

(c) Matching test: In this type of test, the examinee is provided with two lists. In these lists, the subjects are not given in a serially ordered manner. The student expected to serialize them and put them against each other. For example:

1. Dr. Shankar Dayal Sharma	Prime Minister of India
2. P.V. Narasimha Rao	President of India
3. Y.B. Chavan	Finance Minister of India
4. Dr. Man Mohan Singh	Home Minister of India

(d) Classification type of test: In this type of test, the student is given a group of certain words. Out of these words, generally one word is irrelevant. The student is asked to underline that word. For example

Note: Underline the word that is irrelevant.

Uttar Pradesh/Punjab/Haryana/Maharashtra/Bangalore/Kashmir/ Orissa.

2. Recall Type of Test

In this type of test, the power to recall of the student is judged. He is asked to answer the questions that test his recall power. Following are the various types of recall type of test:

1. Simple Recall type of test; and
2. Completion test.

1. *Simple recall type of test:* In this type of test, the students are expected to answer the question on the basis of their memory. Given below is an example of this test:

   (a) When did India get freedom?

(b) Who was the first President of India?

(c) When did Sri Lal Bahadur Shastri die?

2. *Completion test:* In this type of test, the examinees are given incomplete sentences. They are supposed to complete the sentences filling in proper words in the blank places. Given below is an example:

(i) The Prime Minister of India is the leader of the ... party in Parliament.

(ii) The member of Rajya Sabha receive a monthly allowance of Rs. ....

Requirements of the New Type of Test

New type of tests have to be carefully constructed. The following precautions be taken otherwise, these tests are likely to lose the utility:

1. Careful planning and construction.
2. These tests should be carefully planned and constructed only then they shall serve their purpose. For this the following things are needed:

(a) *Determination of the Purpose*. The basic purpose of the test must be decided first.

(b) *Selection of the Test in accordance with the Purpose.* After the purpose has been decided, the test has to be found out which would suit the purpose.

(c) *Objective Questions*. The questions that are constructed should be objective.

(d) *Ability of the Students to be kept in Mind.* The individual differences and the mental ability of the students should be kept in mind, otherwise the purpose shall not be served.

e) *Scoring Key to be Prepared.* The scoring key, that provides answers to the questions, must also be prepared. Unless it is done, the purpose shall not be served. Without this, it shall be difficult to award marks.

(f) *Standardization*. These tests need standardization. Then only it is possible to do away with the element of subjectivity.

(g) *Intelligent Planning.* It is not possible for all the teachers to plan these tests. These tests have to be planned and constructed by intelligent teachers as they require intelligent planning.

Other Types of Tests. In addition to the tests given above, the following types of test are also used:

(a) *Intelligence Test.* The basic objective of these tests is to ascertain the mental capacity or the psychological capacity of the students. These tests require such questions that would give an idea about the mental age of the students.

(b) *Recognition Test.* These tests have the element of the traditional examination as also the new system of examination. In these tests, a figure is drawn or a particular question is given and the students have to recognise it. It may be very easily applied to Geometry.

(c) *Logical Selection Test.* In this test, several names of a particular object are given. The correct and the exact name is to be sorted by the students. This is also a new type of test.

Importance of Blue-print in Constructing Achievement Test

The blue-print here means the plan that the teacher has in evaluating the performance of the pupils.

The blue-print concerns itself to the knowledge acquired by means of study, remembering, thinking, solving problems and formulating hypothesis. It is here that the formulation of instructional objectives and their respective behavioural changes can be clearly identified.

In a blue-print the objectives are listed out horizontally. They are knowledge, understanding, application and skill. Again horizontal forms of test items are indicated. They are essay questions, short answer questions and objective questions.

Vertically we find the content divided into sub-units. The question paper should cover all the sub-units and all the objectives. The score for each type of question viz, essay, short answer and objective type should be fixed.

Dissertation Type of Tests

In this type of examination the examinee has to carry out research work as a prescribed topic. He has also to present dissertation that contains the results of the work done by him. The plan of this work is submitted in writing. In fact, it is an enlarged form of the essay type test.

(iv) Assessment of Regular Work

For such an assessment a record of child's development should be kept. Such a record may be kept for his home-work, practical work etc., and this should be take into consideration while assessing a student.

Thus, we find that no single device is enough and a judicious blend of various evaluation tools is the best approach.

General Suggestions for Constructing Objective Type Tests

The following points be kept in mind while constructing different types of objective tests:

(i) Difficult words and sentences should be avoided.

(ii) Text-book sentences should be avoided.

(iii) Ambiguities should be avoided.

(iv) Clues and suggestions should be avoided.

For **careful planning** and **construction** of such a test following things are needed:

(a) *Determination of the Purpose:* The basic purpose of the test should be decided first.

(b) *Relation of the Test in accordance with the Purpose*: After purpose has been decided, the test has to be found out which would suit the purpose.

(c) *Objective Questions.* The questions that are constructed should be objective.

(d) *Ability of the Student to be kept in Mind.* The individual differences and the mental ability of the students should be kept in mind, otherwise the purpose shall not be served.

(e) *Scoring Key to be Prepared.* The scoring key that provides answer to the questions must be prepared. Unless it is done, the purpose shall not be served. Without it, it shall be different to award marks.

(f) *Standardisations.* These tests need standardisation. Then only it is possible to do away with the element of subjectivity.

(g) *Intelligent Planning.* It is not possible for all the teachers to plan these tests. These tests have to be planned and constructed by intelligent teachers as they require intelligent planning.

While planning these tests following should be avoided:

(i) Difficult words and sentences should be avoided.

(ii) Text-book sentences should be avoided.

REVISION QUESTIONS

1. Giving the meaning and purpose of evaluation, throw light on the importance of evaluation in Social Studies.
2. Discuss the importance of evaluation in Social Studies.
3. What are the defects of existing system of examinations? Give your suggestions for its improvement.
4. How does a new type attainment test differ from traditional test? Illustrate your answer with two types framed on Social Studies syllabus prescribed for any stage of education.

17

Lesson Planning in Social Studies

17.1 INTRODUCTION

A proper planning of lessons is the key to effective teaching. The teacher must know in advance the subject-matter and mode of its delivery in the class-room. This planning will give the teacher idea of how to introduce the topic, how to develop the key concepts, how to correlate the concepts to real life situations and how to conclude the lesson.

According to Bossing, "Lesson plan is the title given to the statement of the achievements to be realised and the specific means by which these are to be attained as a result of the activities engaged in, during the period."

L.B. Stands conceives a lesson plan as "Plan of action" implemented by the teacher in the class-room.

G.H. Green says, "the teacher who has planned his lesson wisely related to his topic and to his class will be in a position to enter the class-room without any anxiety, ready to embark with confidence upon a job he understands and prepared to carry it to a workmanable conclusion. He has far seen the difficulties that are likely to arise, and prepared himself to deal with them. He knows the aims, his lesson is intended to fulfil, and he has marshalled his own resources for the purpose, and because he is free of anxiety, he will be able cooly to estimate the value of his work as the lesson proceeds, equally aware of failure and success and prepared to learn from both."

Though a syllabus is prescribed for each class yet the teacher is at liberty to draw up his own teaching syllabus. It is best to organise the teaching syllabus around a few broad areas of experience of pupils. For this purpose the syllabus is divided into a number of units.

17.2 VALUES AND IMPORTANCE OF LESSON PLANNING

Lesson plan is expected to perform the following functions:

1. Achievement of Definite Goals and Objectives

While preparing his lesson plan the teacher keeps in mind general and specific aims of the lesson. In this way his field of work is delimited and he thinks of various means to achieve these aims.

2. Prevention of Wastage

Planning a lesson helps in avoiding the wastage of time and energy of both the teacher and the taught. A planned lesson will be delivered in a more logical, orderly and systematic way. The main point will never be lost sight of and all efforts will be made to clarify it during the allotted period.

3. Self-confidence on the Part of the Teacher

A teacher who has planned his lesson carefully is full of confidence in his class. He is clear in his mind of the lives on which he has to develop his lecture, which activities are to be undertaken and how to carry his pupils with him. Different steps are clearly explained in his lesson plan and a teacher is therefore sure to achieve success.

4. Thoroughness and Effectiveness

The teacher has spent a lot of energy and time in preparing his lesson plan and he has planned it keeping in view the mental capacitites, attitudes, habits, interests and aptitudes of pupils to be taught. He has tried to make best use of all the available teaching aids and thus it is expected to capture pupils' interests and make learning natural and effective.

5. Evaluation Possible

A good lesson plan enables a teacher to evaluate his work as the lesson proceeds. He will be fully conscious of his success or failure and will try to learn from both, for the future. Evaluation is the most essential part of the teaching-learning process which is possible when definite aims and objectives are kept in view. Learning experiences are given to realise those aims and tests of progress are prepared for judging the outcomes of instructions.

Aims of the Lesson Plan

The lesson plan is expected to show the following things:

(i) The knowledge that the students have acquired.

(ii) The direction towards which the students have to be carried, and the new subject-material that they have to be taught.

(iii) In the beginning we have the general aims and objects of the teaching and in particular, aims and objects of teaching of that subject.

(iv) There is also a statement of experience of the teacher.

(v) It aims at presenting a systematic knowledge of the subject of the students.

Functions of Lesson Plan

Important functions of lesson plan are as follows:

1. It delimits the field of work of the teacher as also of the students and provides a definite objective for each day's work.
2. Since the goal is fixed so teacher gets an impetus to achieve his goal.
3. It prevents the teacher from going off the track.
4. It helps the teacher to organise and systematise the learning process.
5. It helps in avoiding needless repetition.
6. It helps the teacher to overcome the feeling or nervousness and insecurity. It gives him confidence to face the class.
7. It provides opportunity to the teacher to think out new ways and means of making the lesson interesting and to introduce thought provoking questions.
8. It ensures a definite assignment for class and availability of adequate materials for the lesson.

Importance of Herbart in the Field of Lesson Plan

Herbart was the man who introduced this system of Lesson Plan. He was an idealist and believed in imparting education to the students for building up their character. In order to achieve this objective, he gave an important place to the teacher in the educational setup. He gave a general method to be utilised by the teachers for imparting knowledge to the students in the class-room. With the help of this method he could achieve the objective of building of the character of the students.

Four Steps of Herbart

Herbart has laid down the following four steps in his method for teaching. He has said that the Lesson Plan or method of teaching should have the following qualities:

1. Clearness or clarity,
2. Association
3. System, and
4. Method.

Additions of Zillar. Zillar was a disciple of Herbart. He has made an attempt to improve the method of the teaching of Herbart. He has divided the step of clearness into two sub-divisions; namely:

(a) Introduction

(b) Presentation.

Generally, this whole plan is known as five steps of Herbart. This plan of education is said to be very useful in the teaching of Science and Mathematics, but with certain modifications, it can also be utilised for the teaching of other subjects as well. In the following pages we have tried to apply this method in drawing of the lesson plans of social studies.

Features of a Lesson Plan

Some important features of a good lesson plan are as under:

(i) *Objectives*: All the cognitive objectives that are intended to be fulfilled should be listed in the lesson plan.

(ii) *Content*: The subject-matter that is intended to be covered should be limited to prescribed time. The matter must be interesting and it should be related to pupil's previous knowledge. It should also be related to daily life situations.

(iii) *Method(s)*: The most appropriate method be chosen by the teacher. The method chosen should be suitable to the subject matter to be taught. Suitable teaching aids must also be identified by the teacher. Teacher may also use supplementary aids to make his lesson more effective.

(iv) *Evaluation*: Teacher must evaluate his lesson to find the extent to which he has achieved the aim of his lesson. Evaluation can be done even by recapitulation of subject-matter through suitable questions.

17.3 TYPES OF PLANNING

(a) Planning of the work of the year in a definite manner and in unit.

(b) Planning of each unit

(c) Daily lesson planning.

(d) Planning shared with the pupils.

17.4 UNIT PLANNING

A unit is related learning segment made up of a few lessons alongwith an outline of its actual execution in the class-room. Thus a unit will consist of both the subject-matter and methodology of its delivery to students.

Hoover defines units as, "The teaching unit is a group of related concepts from which a given set of instructional and educational experiences is desired. Unit normally range for three to six weeks long."

In view of Preston, a unit is a large chunk or a block of related subject-matter as can be over-viewed by the learner.

After having divided the prescribed syllabus into a number of teaching units the teachers will decide the time that could be allotted to each unit. After that he can break up each unit in a number of lessons and each lesson should be complete in itself. After this the teacher will enter in his diary the scheme of work under the headings.

Some of the advantages of unit planning are as under:

(i) It provides a basic course structure around which specific class activities can be organised.

(ii) It enables the teacher to integrate the basic course concepts and those of related areas into various teaching experiences.

(iii) It provides an opportunity to the teacher to keep a balance between various dimensions of the prescribed course.

Unit No..................................

Date	*Course content*	*Demonstration*	*Equipment material*	*Student's activities*	*Remarks References*

(iv) It enables the teacher to break away from traditional text-book teaching.

If the prescribed course has to be covered in a number of years then it is unitwise to distribute the course in units spread over a number of years.

17.5. STEPS IN LESSON PLANNING (HERBARTIAN STEPS)

Formal steps in lesson planning are:

1. Introduction (or preparation)
2. Presentation
3. Association (or comparison)
4. Generalisation
5. Application
6. Recapitulation.

1. Introduction

It pertains to preparing and motivating children to the lesson content by linking it to the previous knowledge of the student, by arousing curiousity of the children and by making an appeal to their senses. This prepares the child's mind to receive new knowledge. This step though so important must be brief. It may involve testing of previous knowledge of the child. Sometimes the curiosity of pupil can be aroused by some experiment, chart, model, story or even by some useful discussion.

2. Presentation

It involves the stating of the object of lesson and exposure of students to new information. The actual lesson begins and both teacher and students participate. Teacher should make use of different teaching aids to make his lesson effective. Teacher should draw as much as is possible from the students making use of judicious questions. In science lesson it is desirable that a heuristic atmosphere prevails in the class.

3. Association

It is always desirable that new ideas or knowledge be associated to the daily life situations by citing suitable examples and by drawing comparisons with the related concepts. This step is all the more important when we are establishing principles or generalising definitions.

4. Generalisation

In science lessons generally the learning material leads to certain generalisations leading to establishment of certain formulates, principle or laws. An effort be made that the students draw the conclusions themselves. Teacher should guide the students only if their generalisation is either incomplete or irrelevant.

5. Application

In this step of lesson plan the knowledge gained is applied to certain situations. This step is in conformity with the general desire of the students to make use of generalisation in order to see for themselves if the generalisations are valid in certain situations or not? No lesson of science may be considered complete if such rules, principles, formula etc., are not applied to life situations.

6. Recapitulation

In this step of his lesson plan the teacher tries to ascertain whether his students have understood and grasped the subject-matter or not. This is used for assessing the effectiveness of the lesson by asking students questions on the content of the lesson. Recapitulation can also be done by giving a short objective type test to the class or even by asking the students to label some unlabelled sketch.

One most important point to remember is that the six steps given above for lesson planning are formal Herbartian steps and teacher should not try to follow these very rigidly. These are only guidelines and in many a lessons it is not possible to follow all these steps.

There is another way of lesson planning which is gaining currency these days. It is known as *Glover Plan*. This plan has four steps as follows:

1. **Questioning.** Teacher must introduce and develop his lesson through related and sequential questions. Start the lesson by asking questions about previous knowledge of the students. The questions should then lead to new knowledge under consideration.

Lesson can also be introduced with the help of some teaching aid like a picture, chart or model etc., the introduction can also be made by describing a situation or by telling a short story.

However, teacher should bear in mind that the introduction is brief and interesting.

2. Discussion. For discussion the class be divided into smaller groups and in such groups students be encouraged to express their ideas and opinions freely. This helps the students in removal of their difficulties.

3. Investigation. The students are encouraged to do a project or investigation on the lesson topic either individually or in small groups by processing information or by laboratory work.

4. Expression. It concerns the strategy in which the student's and the teacher's communiation of ideas through observation and listening (passive expression) or through doing (active expression) or through fine and performing arts (artistic expression) or by arranging learning situations (organisational expression).

In developing a lesson a teacher must keep in mind the following psychological principles:

(i) *Principle of Selection and Division*. The teacher should wisely select and divide the learning material into smaller segments. It is also for the teacher to decide about the quantum of subject-matter to be covered by him and that which has to be elicited from the students.

(ii) *Principle of Successive Clarity*. It is for the teacher to see that the different learning segments of lesson are well-structured, sequenced and connected. Teacher must ensure, at each segment, that students have grasped the subject-matter given to them.

(iii) *Principle of Integration*. Teacher should conclude his lesson only after combining various learning segments to produce some generalisation.

Design for Writing a Lesson Plan

Lecture-cum-Demonstration Method

The style given below is generally followed for writing a lesson plan:

Class: Date:

Subject: Duration

Topic: of period:

*Instructional Material*______________________________

*General Objectives*______________________________

*Specific Objectives*______________________________

*Previous Knowledge*______________________________

Questions

1. ____________________?
2. ____________________?
3. ____________________?

*Introduction*____________________

*Questions*____________________

1. ____________________?
2. ____________________?

*Announcement of Aim*____________________

____

Presentation

____

Matter	*Method*	*B.B.Summary*

____

*Generalisations*____________________

____

*Applications*____________________

____

*Recapitulation*____________________

*Questions*____________________

1. ____________________?
2. ____________________?
3. ____________________?

*Home Task*____________________

Importance of Black-board Work

For the effective delivery of a lesson a proper use of black-board is a must. The black-board must be used from the beginning of the lesson until its very end. Black-board is the most effective of all the teaching aids. In the teaching of social studies black-board can be used to draw sketches, outlines, diagrams, maps, graphs, pictures, time lines etc. which help to make clear many facts and statements. Black-board can also be used to write down important points. The black-board work throughout the lesson enables pupils to see what they have heard. In this way both the aural and visual sensations are combined and learning is facilitated. It thus is quite clear that in any good lesson plan, black-board work is made an integral part of the plan.

17.6 MODEL LESSON PLAN--1

Class: VI	Date:
Subject: Social Studies	Period: 4th period
Topic: Life of Shivaji	Duation: 40 minutes

General Aims

(i) To inculcate in pupils a sense of patriotism by acquainting them with the great deeds and lives of great men of their country.

(ii) To develop in the students the qualities of chivalry and bravery and to encourage them to become great.

(iii) To develop in students the curiosity to know more and more about social studies.

(iv) To develop in students the right attitudes of fellow feeling, friendliness, co-operation, toleration and international understanding.

Specific Aims

(i) To make students familiar with the life and administration of Shivaji.

(ii) To develop the spirit of patriotism and love for motherland in the students.

Teaching Aids

(i) A full size picture of Shivaji

(ii) A map of India (political) showing the boundaries of the territory under the rule of Shivaji.

Previous Knowledge

Students are already familiar with the names of Lord Rama, Lord Krishna, Ashoka the great etc.

Introduction

The lesson will be introduced by asking the following questions:

(i) Name a few historical personalities born in India.

Ans. Rama, Krishna, Ashoka etc.

(ii) Name the Marahatta personality who struggled hard for keeping India free from English domination.

Not getting a proper reply, the teacher will announce the name of Shivaji and will also announce the topic for the day.

Presentation

Matter	*Method*	*B.B. Summary*
Shivaji was Marahatta Chieftain. He was born in 1627 A.D. Guru Ram Das was taking active part to unite the Marahattas who were willing to lay down their lives for their religion and motherland. Their slogan was, "Destroy the enemy of motherland."	When was Shivaji born?	1627 A.D.
Shivaji was the sun of Shahji who was a courier of Sultan of Ahmed-nagar.	Who was the father of Shivaji?	Shahji
Because of extremely busy life of his father Shivaji was brought up by his mother Jija Bai.	What was the name of Shivaji's mother?	Jija Bai
She told the stories of Ramayana, Mahabharata, etc.	Which stories were narrated to Shivaji by his mother?	Ramayana Mahabharata etc.
These stories made Shivaji a great patriot. He was full of ambitions to defend his motherland.	What effect these stories have on Shivaji?	They made him a great patriot

Recapitulation

The teacher will ask the following questions:

1. When was Shivaji born?
2. What was Shivaji's father?
3. What was the main aim of Marahattas at that time?

Home Work

Write down an outline of the life of Shivaji.

LESSON PLAN--2

Class : X — Time : 40 Minutes

Date : — Period :

Subject : Social Studies — Topic : Place of capital in Industry

General Objectives

(i) To acquaint the students with general principles of economics.

(ii) To explain to students the relationship of Economics with our day-to-day life.

(iii) To teach the students various principles of production, consumption, distribution etc., and to explain their practical importance.

(iv) To develop the economic feeling of students and to make them understand the utility of production.

(v) To acquaint the students with the economic structure of the world.

(vi) To acquaint the students with the ways and means of self-reliance.

Specific Aims

(i) To explain to students the practical utility of capital and wealth.

(ii) To explain to students the important place of the capital and wealth.

Previous Knowledge

Following questions will be asked to test the previous knowledge of the students:

(i) What do you need to purchase something from the market? (Money, rupee etc.)

(ii) Why do you purchase things? (For our use or consumption)

(iii) Can you tell me why is sugar-cane purchased by sugar mills? (Yes, to produce sugar)

(iv) Can you guess the thing that is needed most to produce a thing or commodity? (Yes, capital)

(v) How do you address and name a person who is rich or wealthy? (Capitalist)

(vi) What is the name given to the wealth invested in an industry? (Capital)

Statement of the Aim

At this stage the teacher will announce to the students that today we will study about, "The place of capital in Industry."

Teaching Aids

(i) Black-board, chalk etc.

(ii) Pictures, diagrams and sketches about certain industries.

(iii) Statistics of some industry.

Presentation

Matter	*Method*	*B.B. Summary*
1	2	3
Money is spent to fulfil wants of various types such as personal, business, social etc.	Why is money spent? Name various kinds of need and wants?	To fulfil the wants. Personal, social, business etc.
Various organs of industry are land, capital, labour, management and enterprise. An industrialist purchases land from the land-lord.	Name various organs of an industry	Land, capital, labour, management, enterprise.
He then collects machines and constructs the structures for these machines.	How is land secured by an industrialist?	He purchases land from land-lord by paying him money.
He then arranges for labours and other workers. He pays them wages or salaries in the form of money.	What else is needed by an industrialist to start the industry.	Machines, buildings, workers, raw materials, etc.

1	2	3
He then arranges the raw material and its transport by suitable means of transport (e.g., rail road etc.). He also makes arrangement for transport of finished goods. All this he arranges by paying money.	How does an industrialist manage export, import, transport of raw materials, finished goods etc.?	By using suitable means of transport such as rail, road etc.
Thus, he has to spend money for all his requirements. He spends money to earn profit by running the industry. The industrialist secures the entire profit. Again it is the industrialist who has to bear all the losses and damages if any. This capacity to bear and suffer the loss and earn the profit is called Enterprise. Industrialist or entrepreneur needs capital at every place for procuring and securing all the things needed by him for business.	How does he secure these means? Why does an industrialist spend so much of money ? Who suffers loss and the damage, if any ? What name is given to this capacity to bear and suffer the loss and earn the profit? Name one thing that is needed by industrialist at every place	By spending money. To earn profits. The industrialist Enterprise. Money or Capital.

Recapitulation

Following questions will be asked to recapitulate the lesson:

(i) How is business carried on?

(ii) What is needed most by an industrialist?

(iii) What do you mean by enterprise?

Home-task

Write a short essay on the importance of capital in industry

or

Bring out clearly the importance of land, labour, capital, organisation and enterprise and determine the importance of capital in these things.

LESSON PLAN--3

Class : IX　　Time: 40 Minutes

Date :　　Period :

Subject: Social Studies　　Topic: Localisation of Industries

General Objectives

(i) To acquaint the students with different trades and industries.

(ii) To develop in students the power of thinking and judgement.

(iii) To develop the capacity of students so that they can takke full advantage of the natural resources.

(iv) To explain to students practical aspects and importance of Economic principles.

(v) To develop in students the qualities of cooperation and coordination.

(vi) To equip the students to be able to solve various economic problems.

Specific Aims

To explain to students the underlying principles of localisation of industries.

Previous Knowledge

Following questions will be ased to test the previous knowledge of the students:

(i) Where are the clothes manufactured? (In the mills)

(ii) Where is cement manufactured? (In cement factories)

(iii) Where is sugar prepared? (In sugar factories)

(iv) What is the function of a businessman or an industrialist? (To carry out business and to establish factories)

Statement of Aim

At this stage the teacher will announce to the students that today we will study about "Localisation of the Industries."

Teaching Aids

(i) Black-board, chalk etc.

(ii) Maps depicting the climate; crop, means of communication and transport.

(iii) Figures about the mineral wealth of the country.

Presentation

Matter	*Method*	*B.B. Summary*
A businessman takes up a business to earn profits. For running the business he needs capital. In addition to this he needs workers, machiens, raw materials etc. He needs a competent manager to look after his business and to advise him in its expansion etc. Duties of manager are multifarious and include everything about the industry. He is expected to make all the arrangements and at minimum expenses in [illegible]test possible time. He is [illegible]e into consideration [illegible]s such as the avoid-[illegible]ility of raw materials, labours, means of transport etc.	What for is business carried out?	To earn profit
	Which thing is needed most to run any business?	Money or capital
	List a few important duties of a manager	1. To arrange for labour materials. 2. To arrange for labour. 3. To arrange for transport of raw material. 4. To make cost analysys of various options available. 5. To arrange to sell finished goods.
	Name some factors which should be given due consideration while setting up an industry	1. Cheap labour and raw material should be available. 2. Transportation is easy. 3. Climate is suitable

Recapitulation

Folowing questions will be asked to recapitulate the lesson:

(i) What are the functions of a manager in a mill?

(ii) What is the importance of the suitability of the location for any industry?

(iii) What sort of place be needed for running textile industry?

Home-task

Indicate, with reasons, a place that would be suitable for setting up a wood industry.

REVISION QUESTIONS

1. Describe briefly the things that are required for drawing a lesson-plan.
2. What is the importance of lesson planning in the teaching of social studies? Give an outline of a lesson plan in Social Studies.
3. Discuss the aims and objectives of a lesson plan.
4. Draw a general proforma of a lesson plan.
5. Give five Herbartian steps of a lesson plan.